Virtual Clinical Excursions—Medical-Surgical

for

Potter & Perry: FUNDAMENTALS OF NURSING, 6th Edition

prepared by

Patricia A. Potter, RN, MSN, PhD, CMAC, FAAN

Virtual Clinical Excursions CD-ROM prepared by

Jay Shiro Tashiro, PhD, RN
Director of Systems Design
Wolfsong Informatics
Sedona, Arizona

Gina Long, RN, DNSc
Assistant Professor, Department of Nursing
College of Health Professions
Northern Arizona University
Flagstaff, Arizona

Ellen Sullins, PhD
Director of Research
Wolfsong Informatics
Sedona, Arizona

Michael Kelly, MS
Director of the Center for Research and
Evaluation of Advanced Technologies
in Education
Northern Arizona University
Flagstaff, Arizona

The development of Virtual Clinical Excursions Volume 1 was partially funded by the National Science Foundation, under grant DUE 9950613.
Principal investigators were Tashiro, Sullins, Long, and Kelly.

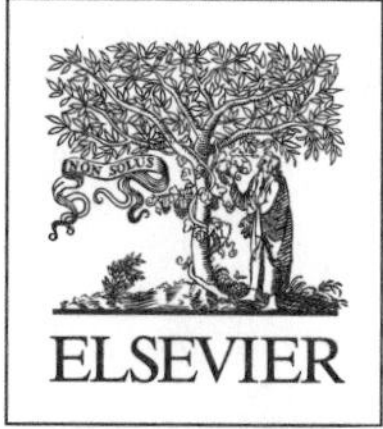

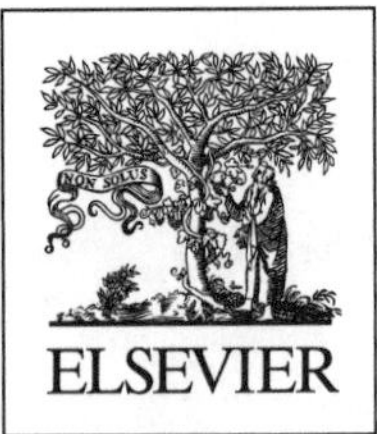

11830 Westline Industrial Dr.
St. Louis, Missouri 63146

VIRTUAL CLINICAL EXCURSIONS FOR POTTER & PERRY: FUNDAMENTALS OF NURSING, 6TH EDITION
ISBN 0-323-03001-7

Notice

Nursing is an ever-changing field. Standard safety precautions must be followed, but as new research and clinical experience broaden our knowledge, changes in treatment and drug therapy may become necessary or appropriate. Readers are advised to check the most current product information provided by the manufacturer of each drug to be administered to verify the recommended dose, the method and duration of administration, and contraindications. It is the responsibility of the licensed prescriber, relying on experience and knowledge of the patient, to determine dosages and the best treatment for each individual patient. Neither the publisher nor the editor assumes any liability for any injury and/or damage to persons or property arising from this publication.

The Publisher

First Edition 2003. Second Edition 2005.

Senior Editor: *Tom Wilhelm*
Senior Developmental Editor: *Jeff Downing*
Associate Developmental Editor: *Jennifer Anderson*
Project Manager: *Gayle May*
Designer: *Wordbench*
Cover Art: *Kathi Gosche*

WB/EB

Printed in the United States of America

Last digit is the print number: 9 8 7 6 5 4 3 2 1

Workbook
prepared by

Patricia A. Potter, RN, MSN, PhD, CMAC, FAAN
Research Scientist
Barnes-Jewish Hospital
St. Louis, Missouri

Textbook

Patricia A. Potter, RN, MSN, PhD, CMAC, FAAN
Research Scientist
Barnes-Jewish Hospital
St. Louis, Missouri

Anne Griffin Perry, RN, MSN, EdD, FAAN
Professor and Interim Director of Research
Saint Louis University School of Nursing
Saint Louis University Health Sciences Center
St. Louis, Missouri

Contents

Table of Contents—Potter, Perry: Fundamentals of Nursing, 6th edition

Getting Started

GETTING SET UP

■ MINIMUM SYSTEM REQUIREMENTS

Virtual Clinical Excursions—Medical-Surgical is a hybrid CD, so it runs on both Macintosh and Windows platforms. To use *Virtual Clinical Excursions—Medical-Surgical*, you will need one of the following systems:

- **Windows™**

  Windows 2000, 98SE, ME, XP
  IBM compatible computer
  Pentium II processor (or equivalent)
  300 MHz
  96 MB
  800 × 600 screen size
  Thousands of colors
  100 MB hard drive space
  12× CD-ROM drive
  Soundblaster 16 soundcard compatibility
  Stereo speakers or headphones

- **Macintosh®**

  MAC OS 10.2 or 10.3
  Apple Power PC G3
  300 MHz
  128 MB
  800 × 600 screen size
  Thousands of colors
  100 MB hard drive space
  12× CD-ROM drive
  Stereo speakers or headphones

Ideally, the system you use should have at least 200 MB of free disk space on your hard drive. There are commercially available desktop utility programs that can help clean up your hard drive. No other applications besides the operating system should be running at the time *Virtual Clinical Excursions—Medical-Surgical* is running.

INSTALLING *VIRTUAL CLINICAL EXCURSIONS—MEDICAL-SURGICAL*

- **Windows™**

1. Start Microsoft Windows and insert *Virtual Clinical Excursions—Medical-Surgical* **Disk 1** in the CD-ROM drive.
2. Click the **Start** button on the taskbar and select the **Run** option.
3. Type d:\Windows 95 setup.exe or d:\Windows 98-XP setup.exe (depending on your operating system—where "d:\" is your CD-ROM drive) and press **OK**.
4. Follow the on-screen instructions for installation.
5. Remove *Virtual Clinical Excursions—Medical-Surgical* **Disk 1** from your CD-ROM drive.
6. Restart your computer.

- **Macintosh®**

1. Insert *Virtual Clinical Excursions—Medical-Surgical* **Disk 1** in the CD-ROM drive. The disk icon will appear on your desktop.
2. Double-click on the disk icon.
3. Double-click on the icon that reads **Install Virtual Clinical Excursions**.
4. Follow the on-screen instructions for installation.
5. Remove *Virtual Clinical Excursions—Medical-Surgical* **Disk 1** from your CD-ROM drive.
6. Restart your computer.

HOW TO ADJUST YOUR MONITOR'S SETTINGS (WINDOWS™ ONLY)

- **Windows 95/98/SE/ME/2000**

1. Click the **Start** button and go to **Settings** on the pop-up menu. Click on **Control Panel**.
2. When the Control Panel window opens, double-click on the **Display** icon.
3. You will now be presented with the Display Properties window. Click on the **Settings** tab (on the right). Below the image of the monitor, you will see on the left the **Color** palette. (You should change this to **High Color [16 bit]** by selecting it from the drop-down menu. You will need to restart your computer to do this.) On the right is the desktop area. Left-click and hold down on the slider button and move it to 800 by 600 pixels. Now click **OK**.
4. Windows will ask you to confirm the change; click **OK**. Your screen will resize and Windows will again ask you whether you want to keep these new settings. Click **Yes**.

- **Windows XP**

1. Click the **Start** button; then click **Control Panel** on the pop-up menu.
2. Click **Display**. If Display does not appear, click **Switch to Classic View**; then click on **Display** icon.
3. From the Display Properties dialog box, select the **Settings** tab.
4. Under Screen Resolution, click and drag the sliding bar to adjust the desktop size to 800 x 600 pixels.
5. Under Color Quality, choose **High** or **Highest**.
6. Click **Apply**. If you approve of the new settings, click **Yes**.

HOW TO ACCESS PATIENTS

Unlike previous VCE products that presented all of the patients on one disk, *Virtual Clinical Excursions—Medical-Surgical* includes patients on both disks. Both of the patients in the Intensive Care Unit (Floor 5) are found on Disk 1, which you used to install the program. The remaining patients—including four patients in the Medical-Surgical-Telemetry Unit (Floor 6) and one patient who spends time in the Medical-Surgical-Telemetry Unit (Floor 6) and in the Surgery Department (Floor 4)—are located on Disk 2. When you want to work with any of the seven patients in the virtual hospital, follow these steps:

- **Windows™**
  1. Insert the *Virtual Clinical Excursions—Medical-Surgical* disk that contains the patient you want to work with into your CD-ROM drive.
  2. Double-click on the icon **Shortcut to Virtual Clinical Excursions**, which can be found on your desktop. This will load and run the program.
- **Macintosh®**
  1. Insert the *Virtual Clinical Excursions—Medical-Surgical* disk that contains the patient you want to work with into your CD-ROM drive.
  2. Double-click on the icon **Shortcut to Virtual Clinical Excursions**, which can be found on your desktop. This will load and run the program.

QUALITY OF VISUALS, SPEED, AND COMMON PROBLEMS

Virtual Clinical Excursions—Medical-Surgical uses the Apple QuickTime media layer system. This includes QuickTime Video and QuickTime VR Video, which allow for high-quality graphics and digital video. The graphics seen in the *Virtual Clinical Excursions—Medical-Surgical* courseware should be of high quality with rich color. If the movies and graphics appear blocky or grainy, check to see whether your video card is set to "thousands of colors."

Note: Virtual Clinical Excursions—Medical-Surgical is not designed to function at a 256-color depth. To adjust your monitor's settings, see instructions on p. 2.

The system should respond quickly and smoothly. In particular, you should not see any jerky motions or experience unusual delays as you move through the virtual hospital settings, interact with patients, or access information resources. If you notice slow, jerky, or delayed software responses, it may mean that your particular system requires additional RAM, your processor does not meet the basic requirements, or your hard drive is full or too fragmented. If the videos appear banded or subject to "breakup," you may need to find an updated video driver for the computer's video card. Please consult the manufacturer of the video card or computer for additional video drivers for your machine.

If you are experiencing misplacement of text or cursors in the Electronic Patient Record (EPR), it is likely that your computer operating system has enabled font smoothing. Please turn font smoothing off by following these instructions:

- **Windows™**

  From the Control Panel window click on **Display** and then select the **Appearance** tab. Click on **Effects** and make sure the box next to "Smooth Edges of Screen Fonts" option is unselected.

- **Macintosh®**

  From the desktop, click on the **Apple** icon in the upper left corner. From the drop-down menu, select **Control Panel**; then select **Appearance**. Click on the **Fonts** tab and make sure the selection box next to "Smooth all fonts on screen" is unselected.

Virtual Clinical Excursions—Medical-Surgical uses Adobe Acrobat Reader version 5 to display information in certain places in the simulation. If you cannot see any information when accessing the Charts, Medication Administration Record (MAR), or Kardex, it is likely that Adobe Acrobat Reader was not installed properly when you installed *Virtual Clinical Excursions—Medical-Surgical*. To remedy this, you can manually install Acrobat Reader from the *Virtual Clinical Excursions—Medical-Surgical* **Disk 1**. Double-click the **Adobe Acrobat Reader** installer (ar505enu.exe) on the disk and follow the on-screen instructions. Once the installer has finished installing Acrobat Reader, restart your computer and then resume your use of *Virtual Clinical Excursions—Medical-Surgical*.

TECHNICAL SUPPORT

Technical support for this product is available at no charge by calling the Technical Support Hotline between 9 a.m. and 5 p.m. (Central Time), Monday through Friday. Inside the United States, call 1-800-692-9010. Outside the United States, call 314-872-8370.

Trademarks: Windows™ is a registered trademark.

A QUICK TOUR

Welcome to *Virtual Clinical Excursions—Medical-Surgical*, a virtual hospital setting in which you can work with seven patient simulations and also learn to access and evaluate the health information resources that are essential for high-quality patient care.

The virtual hospital, **Canyon View Regional Medical Center**, is a multistory teaching hospital with a Well-Child Clinic, Pediatric Floor, Surgery Department, Intensive Care Unit, and a Medical-Surgical Floor with a Telemetry Unit. You will have access to the adult patients in the Intensive Care Unit and on the Medical-Surgical Floor. One patient will also spend time in the Surgery Department, where you can follow her through a perioperative experience.

Although each floor plan in the medical center is different, each is based on a realistic hospital architecture modeled from a composite of several hospital settings. All floors have:

- A Nurses' Station
- Patients, seen either in examination areas or in their inpatient rooms
- Patient records, including a Chart, Kardex plan of care, Medication Administration Record, and Electronic Patient Record accessed through a simulated computerized system.

BEFORE YOU START

When you use *Virtual Clinical Excursions—Medical-Surgical*, make sure you have your text-book nearby to consult topic areas as needed. Also make sure that you have both disks to run the simulations. If you have not already installed your *VCE—Medical-Surgical* software, do so now by following the steps outlined in **Getting Set Up** at the beginning of this workbook.

ENTERING THE HOSPITAL AND SELECTING A CLINICAL ROTATION

To begin your tour of Canyon View Regional Medical Center, insert your *Virtual Clinical Excursions—Medical-Surgical* Disk 2 and double-click on the desktop icon **Shortcut to VCE—Medical-Surgical**. Wait for the hospital entrance screen to appear (see below). This is your signal that the program is ready to run. Your first task is to get to the unit where you will be caring for patients and to let someone know when you arrive at the unit. As in any multistory hospital, you will enter the hospital lobby area, take an elevator to your assigned unit, and sign in at the Nurses' Station.

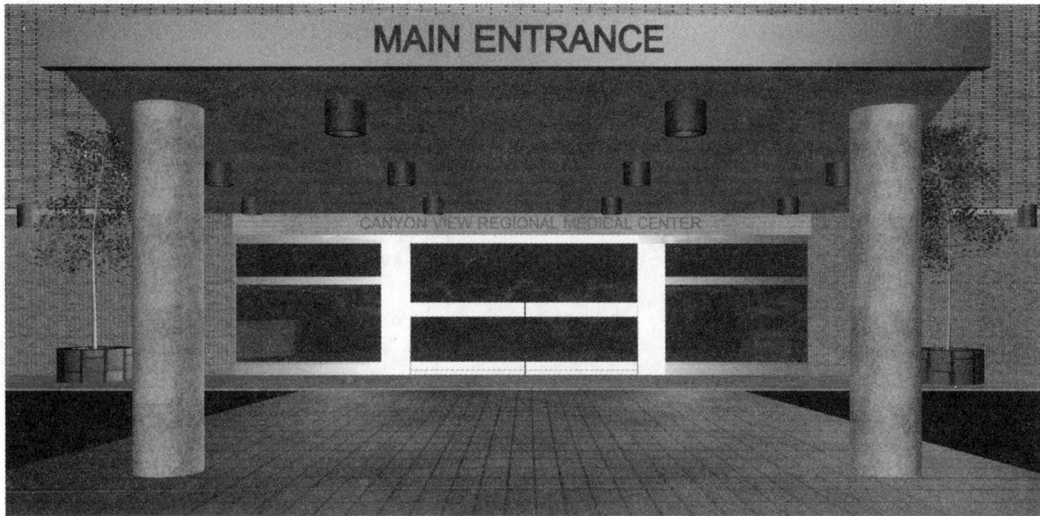

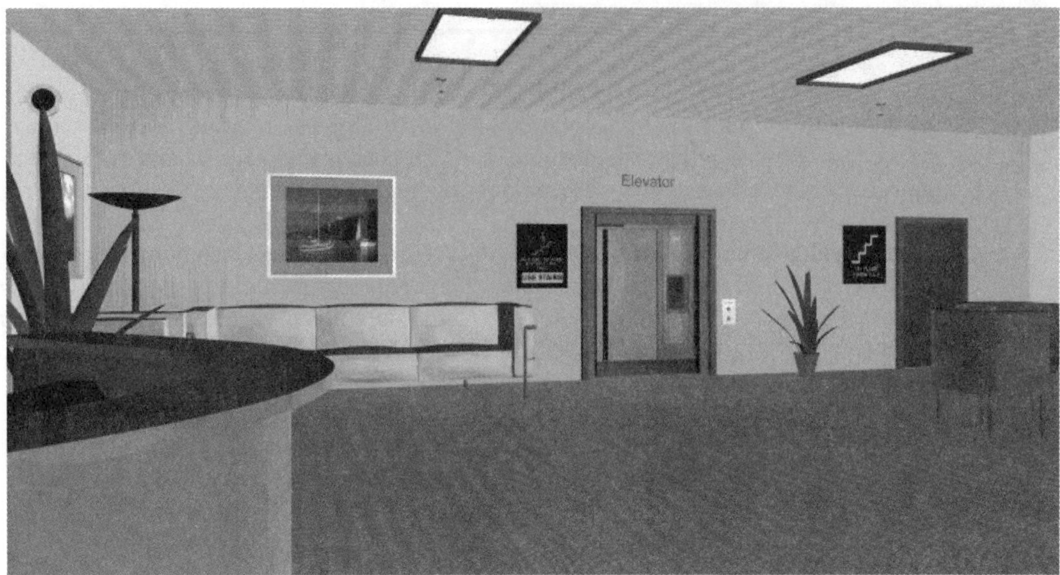

Let's practice getting to your unit in Canyon View Regional Medical Center by following this sequence:

- Click on the hospital entrance door and you will find yourself in the hospital lobby on the first floor (see above).
- Across the lobby, you will see an elevator with a blinking red light. Click on the open doorway and you will be transported into the elevator (see below).
- Now click on the panel on the right side of the doorway. The panel will expand to reveal buttons that allow you to go to the other floors of the hospital (see p. 7).
- Slowly run your cursor across the buttons to familiarize yourself with the different floors and units of the hospital.

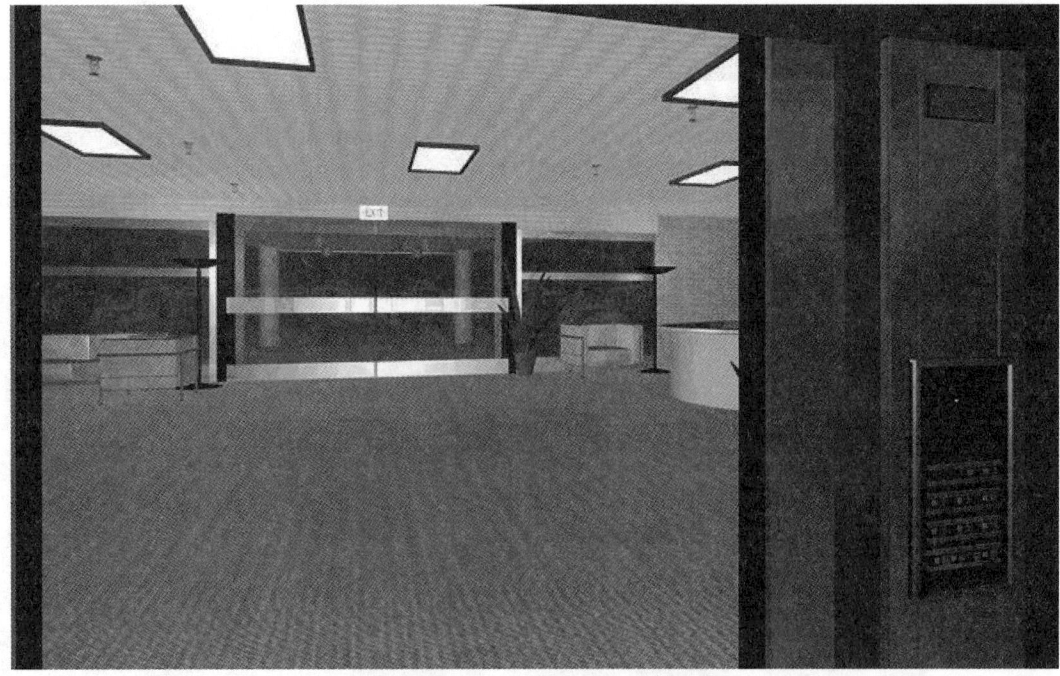

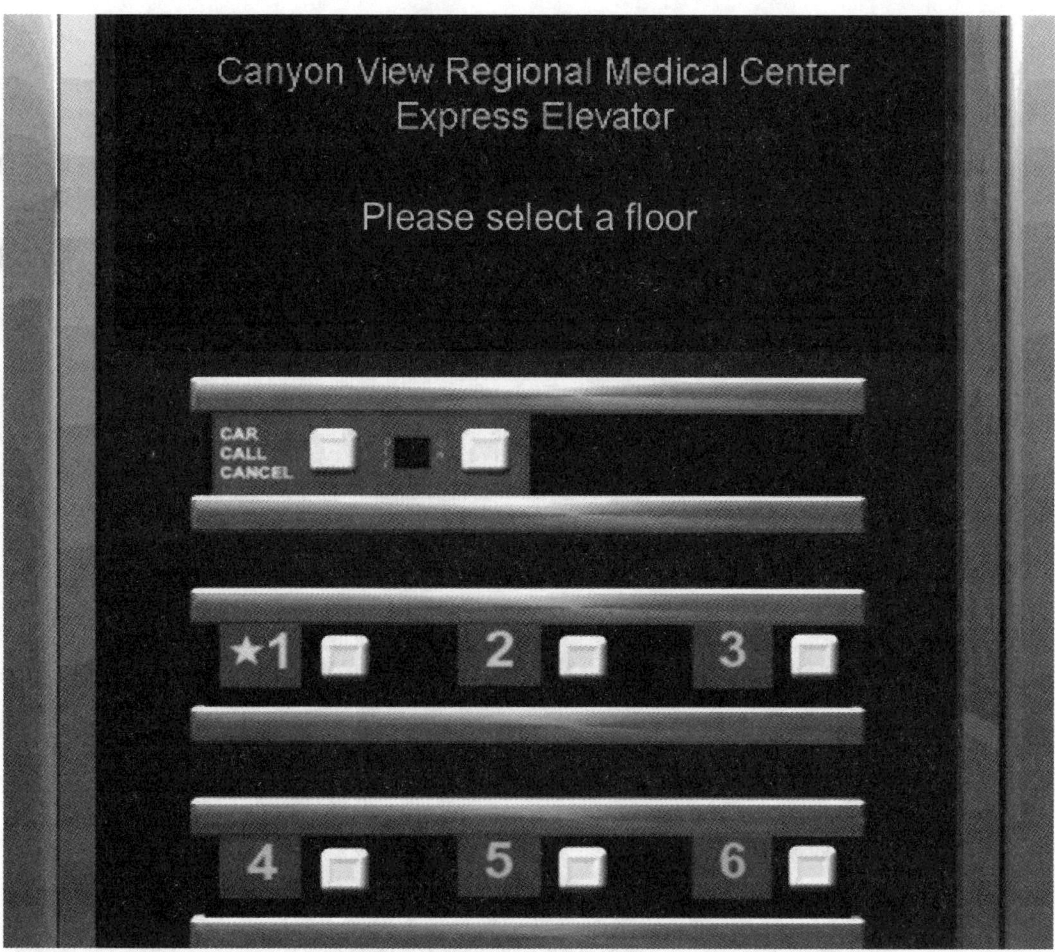

Since you are in a medical-surgical rotation, you will not be able to visit the Well-Child Clinic or the Pediatric Floor. However, you can work with two patients in the Intensive Care Unit (Disk 1), four patients on the Medical-Surgical/Telemetry Floor (Disk 2), and one who spends time on both the Medical-Surgical/Telemetry Floor and in the Surgery Department (Disk 2).

Now, go to a unit and sign in for patient care. With Disk 2 in your CD-ROM drive, try this:

- Click on the button for the Medical-Surgical/Telemetry Floor, which is Floor 6.
- The elevator takes you to that floor and opens onto a virtual unit with a Nurses' Station in the center and rooms arrayed around the Nurses' Station.
- Click on the **Nurses' Station** and you will be transported behind its counter.
- If you click and hold the mouse button down, you can get a 360° view of the Medical-Surgical/Telemetry floor by dragging your mouse left or right. With the button still held down, drag to the left, then up, then down. You get a complete view of the Nurses' Station and the floor (see p. 8).
- Take a few minutes to familiarize yourself with the Nurses' Station. Find the two computers, one of which has **Login** on its screen. This is the computer that allows you to select a patient. The other computer is the **Electronic Patient Records** terminal. As you look around the Nurses' Station, you also will see the patient Charts, the Kardex plan of care notebooks, and the Medication Administration Record notebook (labeled MAR).

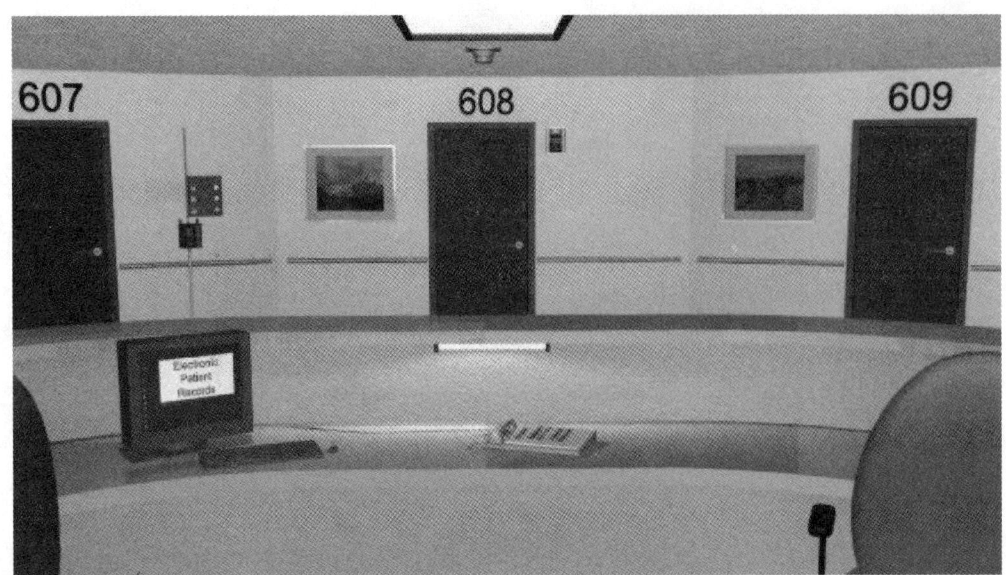
607
608
609
Electronic Patient Records

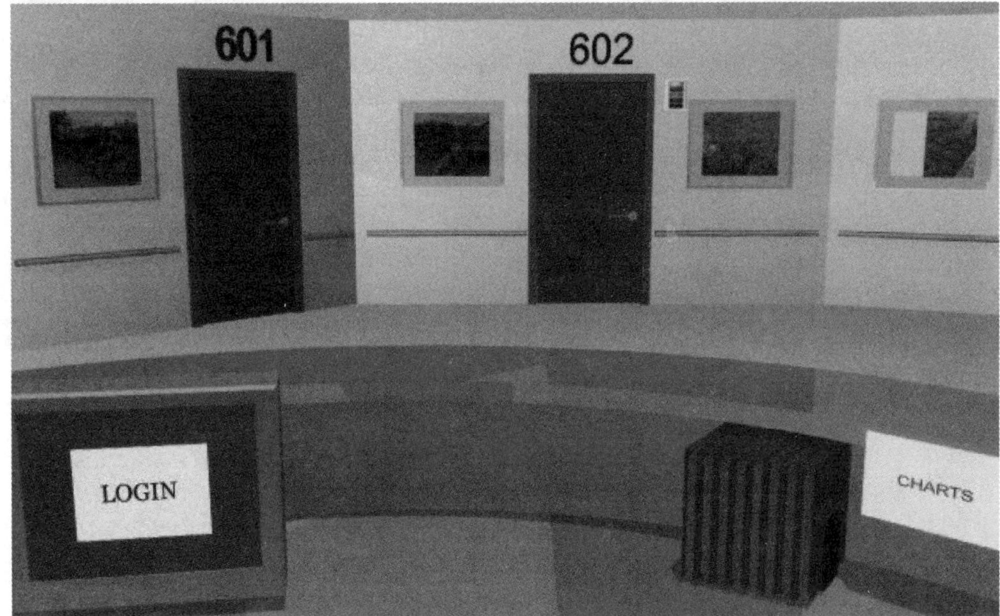
601
602
LOGIN
CHARTS

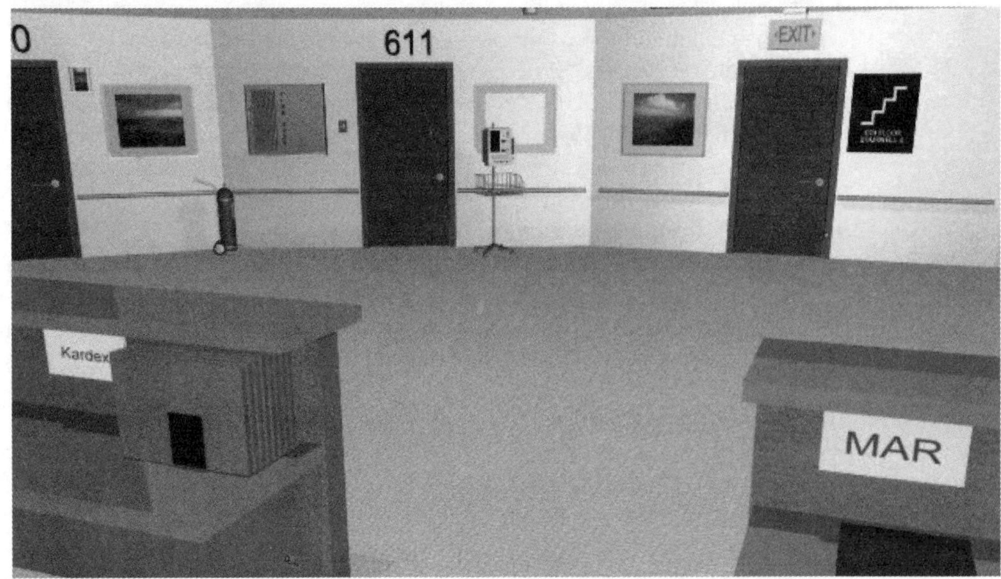
611
EXIT
Kardex
MAR

WORKING WITH PATIENTS

In *Virtual Clinical Excursions—Medical-Surgical*, the Medical-Surgical/Telemetry floor can be visited between 07:00 and 15:00, but a user can see only one patient at a time and then only in blocks of time. We call these blocks "periods of care." In any of the Medical-Surgical/Telemetry floor scenarios, you can select a patient and a period of care by accessing the Supervisor's (Login) Computer. Double-click on this computer to open the sign-in screen, which contains a box with instructions. Click the **Login** button and you will see a screen that lists the patients on this floor and the periods of care in which you can visit and work with them. Again, only one patient can be selected at a time. When work is completed on that patient, you can select another period of care for that patient or another patient.

Note: During a patient simulation you may receive an on-screen message informing you that the current period of care has ended. If this occurs and you have not yet completed the assigned activities (or if you want to review part of the simulation), you can return to the Supervisor's Computer and sign in again for the same patient and period of care. When the Warning screen appears, click **Erase**. On the other hand, if you simply want to review the data you entered during that period of care, you can sign in for the same patient in a later time period and review data in the EPR. Please note that this option doesn't apply to the final period of care. If you are working with a patient during the last period of care, make sure you keep an eye on the on-screen clock and are aware of how much time is remaining.

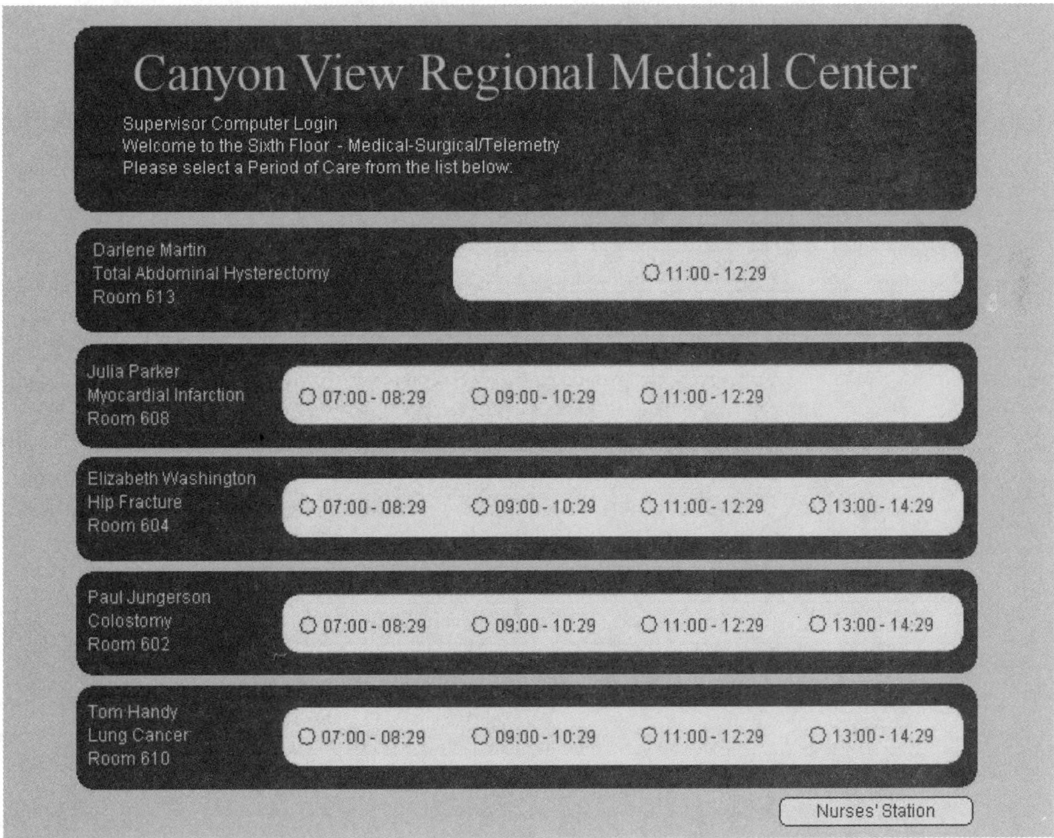

You can choose any of the five patients on this floor (but only one at a time). For each patient you will select a period of care. Four of the patients (Julia Parker, Elizabeth Washington, Paul Jungerson, and Tom Handy) can be seen during four periods of care: 07:00–08:29, 09:00–10:29, 11:00–12:29, and 13:00–14:29. You will follow the fifth patient, Darlene Martin, through a Perioperative Rotation. You see her first in the Surgery Department (Floor 4) for a Preoperative Interview (conducted two days prior to surgery). She then goes to the Surgery Department for preoperative care, surgery, and a period in the PACU (09:30–10:29). After leaving PACU, she is transferred to the Medical-Surgical/Telemetry Floor (Floor 6) at 11:00, and you can see her on that floor from 11:00–12:29.

There are two patients (James Story and James Franklin) in the Intensive Care Unit. Although the patients in the Surgery Department (Floor 4) and the Medical-Surgical/Telemetry Floor (Floor 6) are all found on Disk 2, the patients in the ICU are found on Disk 1. Here are the steps to follow when you need to swap disks:

- If you are currently signed in for a patient, go to the Supervisor's (Login) Computer and sign out. Return to the Nurses' Station.
- Leave the Nurses' Station and enter the elevator. Once you are inside the elevator, remove the disk from your CD-ROM drive and replace it with the other disk.
- Click on the button of the floor number where you need to go.

If you attempt to access the Intensive Care Unit (Floor 5) while Disk 2 is in your CD-ROM drive, the computer will eject the disk and prompt you to insert Disk 1 to continue (see below). Likewise, if you attempt to access the Surgery Department or the Medical-Surgical/Telemetry Floor while Disk 1 is in your CD-ROM drive, the disk will be ejected and the computer will prompt you to insert Disk 2 to continue.

(*Note:* The process of selecting patients is basically the same on all floors of Canyon View Regional Medical Center, although the available periods of care in the Surgery Department are different from those in Medical-Surgical/Telemetry Floor and the Intensive Care Unit. You will observe this when you visit the other floors.)

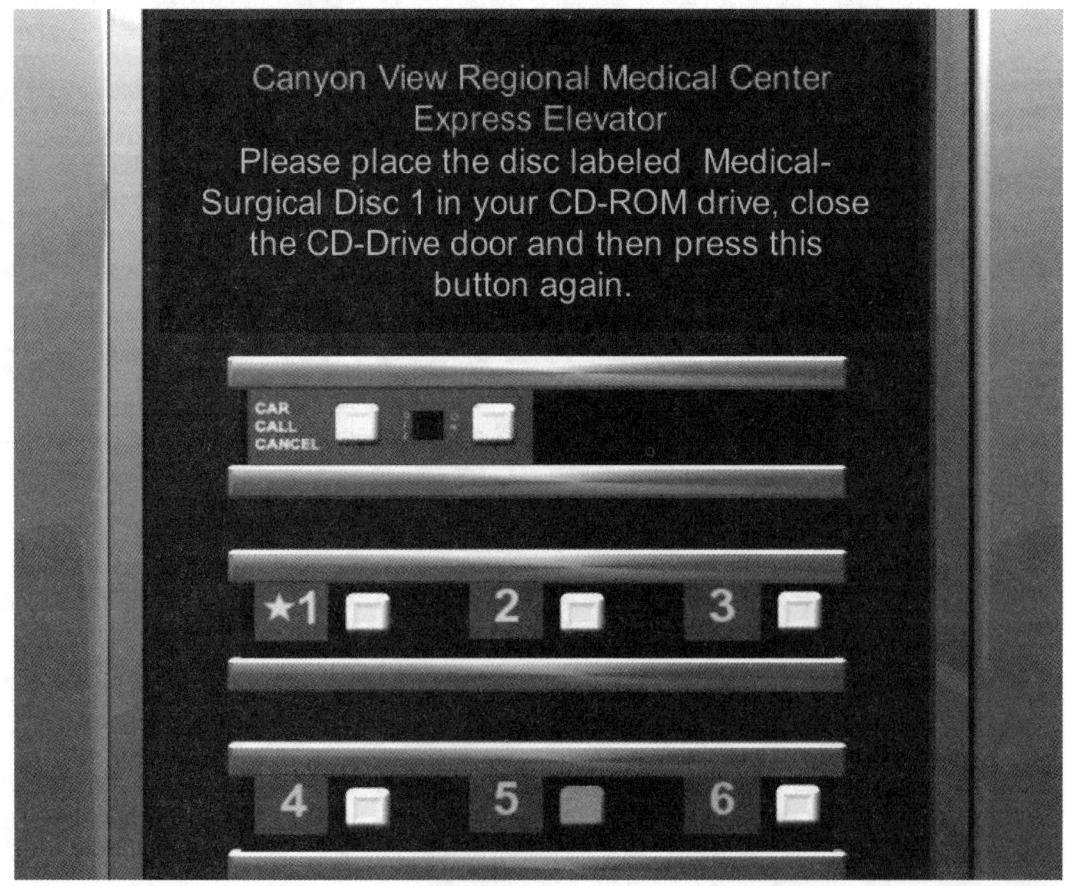

PATIENT LIST

◆ Floor 4: Surgery Department (Disk 2)

- Darlene Martin
  Ms. Martin is a 49-year-old female who begins Tuesday in the Surgery Department to prepare for a total abdominal hysterectomy. She has been suffering from irregular periods and an enlarged uterus over the past six months, which has caused endometrial hyperplasia. A few days before her surgery, she had a preoperative interview. On Tuesday morning she enters a period of preoperative care, then undergoes a hysterectomy. After a period in the Post-Anesthesia Care Unit (PACU), she is transferred to the Medical-Surgical/Telemetry Floor.

◆ Floor 5: Intensive Care Unit (Disk 1)

- James Franklin (Room 504)
  Mr. Franklin is a 67-year-old male who was admitted for a right carotid endarterectomy. Before admission, he experienced five or six episodes of transient left arm and left leg numbness and weakness and one episode of transient expressive aphasia.

- James Story (Room 512)
  Mr. Story is a 42-year-old male who arrived in the Emergency Department complaining of shortness of breath, increasing weakness with a tingling sensation in his extremities, nausea, recent onset of diarrhea, lower leg edema, and a significantly edematous right arm. Mr. Story has type 1 (insulin-dependent) diabetes mellitus and has been undergoing hemodialysis treatment for almost a year. During his stay, he begins experiencing renal failure.

◆ Floor 6: Medical-Surgical/Telemetry Floor (Disk 2)

- Paul Jungerson (Room 602)
  Mr. Jungerson is a 61-year-old male who is recovering from a colon resection. He has a history of diverticulitis, hypertension, pneumonia, and chronic ankle pain.

- Elizabeth Washington (Room 604)
  Ms. Washington is a 63-year-old female who was admitted following an auto accident in which she fractured her hip. She has a history of hypertension and asthma.

- Julia Parker (Room 608)
  Ms. Parker is a 51-year-old female who presented to the Emergency Department with indigestion and mid-back pain. She has a history of hypertension, type 2 diabetes, hyperlipidemia, and obesity. During her stay, she undergoes a heart catheterization and angioplasty, before suffering a myocardial infarction.

- Tom Handy (Room 610)
  Mr. Handy is a 62-year-old male who was admitted 3 days ago for a lobectomy, after being diagnosed with squamous cell carcinoma of the right lung. A long-time smoker, he has a history of chronic bronchitis and benign prostatic hyperplasia.

- Darlene Martin (Room 613)
  Remember Darlene Martin, the surgical patient? (See Floor 4 above.) After a period in the PACU, Ms. Martin is transferred to the Medical-Surgical/Telemetry Floor.

VISITING A PATIENT

Each time you sign in for a new patient and period of care, you enter the simulation at the start of that period of care. The simulations are constructed so that you can conduct a fairly complete assessment of your patient in the first 30 minutes of each period of care. However, after completing a general survey, you should begin to focus your assessments on specific areas. For example, within one period of care you should not do a head-to-toe examination each time you come into a patient's room. Instead, conduct a complete physical at the start of a period of care, then select assessments that are appropriate for your patient's current condition and are based on how that condition is changing. Just as in the real world, a patient's data will change over time as the patient improves or deteriorates. Even if a patient remains stable, there will be diurnal variations in physiology, and these will be reflected in changes in assessment data.

As soon as you sign in to begin working with a patient, a clock appears on screen to help you keep track of time. The clock, which operates in "real time," is located in the bottom left-hand corner of the screen when you are in the Nurses' Station and in the top right-hand corner when you are in the patient's room.

To become familiar with some of the learning resources in *Virtual Clinical Excursions—Medical-Surgical*, insert Disk 2 in your CD-ROM drive, go to Floor 6, select Elizabeth Washington, and choose the 07:00–08:29 period of care. Then click on the button in the lower right corner labeled **Nurses' Station**. This procedure will select the patient and time period for your work. You are then automatically sent to a Case Overview, which provides a short video in which your preceptor introduces the patient. There is also a button labeled **Assignment**. Clicking on this button will open a summary sheet that provides information about the patient and guidance for your work in the simulation.

After completing the Case Overview, you can enter the simulation by clicking on the **Nurses' Station** button in the lower right corner of the screen. This will take you back to the Nurses' Station, where you can begin working with your patient. Remember three things:

- You must select a patient and period of care before any of that patient's simulation and data become available to you.
- Just as in the real world, the Nurses' Station is the base from which you can access patient records and from which you go onto the floor to visit a patient.
- Before you can access another patient simulation, you must go back to the Supervisor's (Login) Computer and follow the procedure to sign out from your current period of care.

Now that you have signed in to care for a patient, Elizabeth Washington, you have several choices. You can enter Elizabeth's room and work with your preceptor to assess the patient. You can review her patient records, which include her Chart, a Kardex plan of care, her active Medication Administration Record (MAR), or the Electronic Patient Record (EPR), all of which contain data that have been collected since Elizabeth entered the hospital. You may know that some hospitals have only paper records and others have only electronic records. Canyon View Regional Medical Center, the virtual hospital, has a combination of paper records (the patient's Chart, Kardex, and MAR) and electronic records (the EPR).

Let's begin by becoming more familiar with the Nurses' Station screen. In the upper left-hand corner, find a menu with these five buttons:

- Patient Care
- Planning Care
- Patient Records
- Case Conference
- Clinical Review

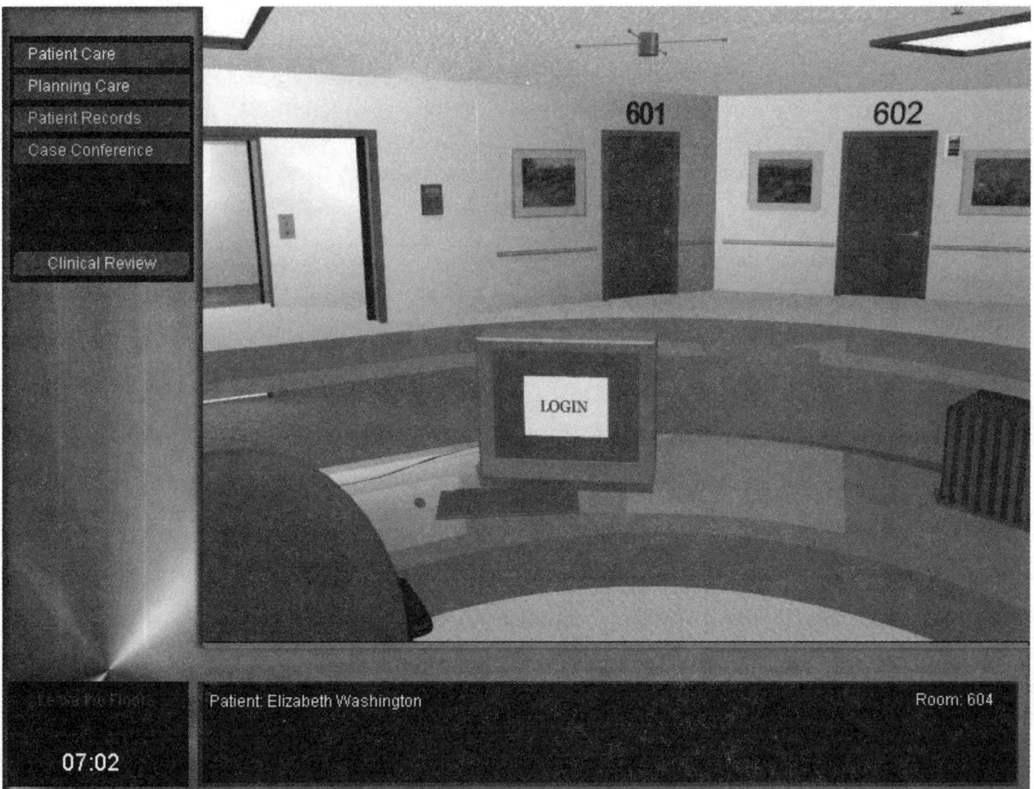

One at a time, single-click on these buttons to reveal drop-down menus with additional options for each item. First, click on **Patient Care**. Two options are available for this item: **Case Overview** and **Data Collection**. You completed the Case Overview after signing in for Ms. Washington, but you can always go back to review it. For example, you might want to return there and click the **Assignment** button to review the summary of Ms. Washington's care up to the start of your shift—or to remind yourself what tasks you have been asked to complete.

◆ Data Collection

To conduct an assessment of your patient, click **Patient Care** and then **Data Collection** from the drop-down menu. This will take you into a small anteroom (part of the patient's room) with a sink, laundry bin, and biohazards waste receptacle. *Note:* You can also enter this anteroom by clicking on the outer door of Ms. Washington's room (Room 604). To visit your patient, complete these steps:

- First *wash your hands!* Click on the sink once to indicate you are beginning to wash. Click again to indicate you are finished washing.
- Now click on the curtain to the right of the sink and enter the patient's room.

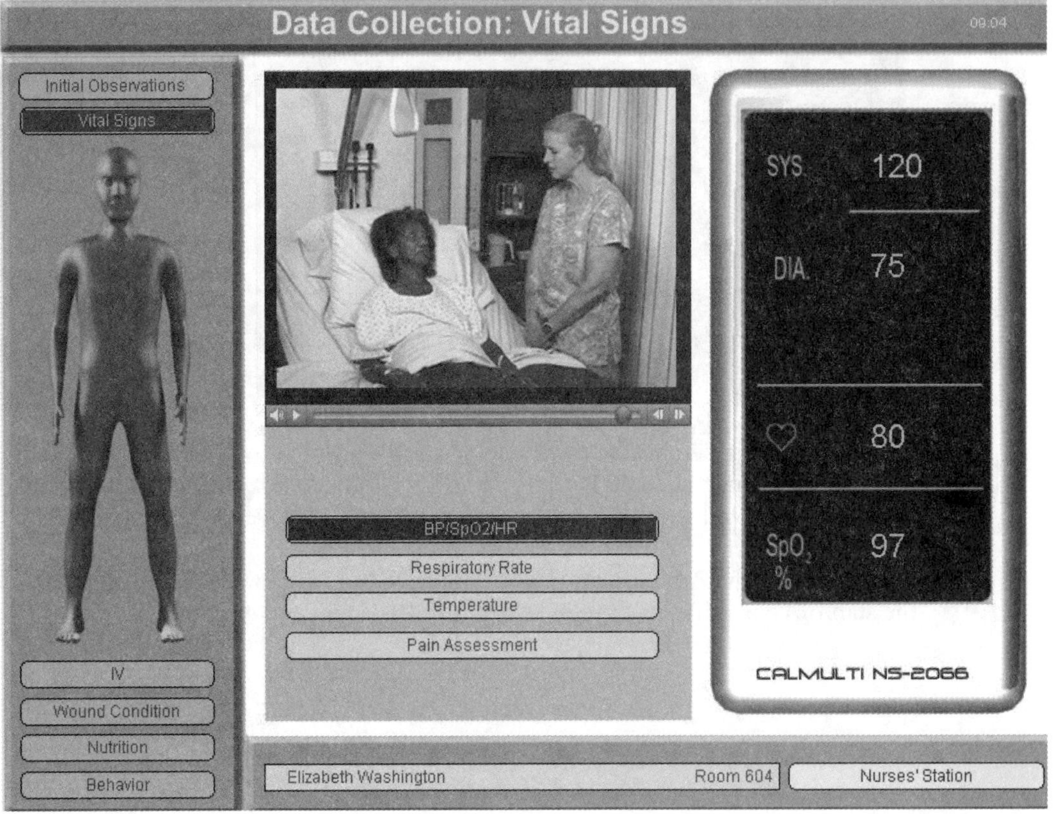

Once in the patient's room, your screen is equipped with various tools you can use for data collection. In the center of the screen, you will see a still frame of your patient. Along the left side of the screen are buttons and a body model that allow you to access learning activities in which your preceptor conducts different types of assessments. Try clicking on the buttons and different body parts. (Note that the body model rotates once your cursor touches it. As you move your cursor over the model, various body parts are highlighted in orange.)

What happened when you clicked on the buttons or body parts? Many of the buttons open options for additional assessments—these always appear below the video screen. Likewise, clicking on a highlighted area of the body model opens options for additional assessments. The body model serves two purposes. First, it provides a way for you to develop a sense of what assessments and physiologic systems are associated with different areas of the human body. Second, it acts as a quick navigational tool that allows you to focus on certain types of assessments.

Note that the body model is a "generic" figure without specific sexual or racial characteristics. However, we encourage you to always think about your patients as unique individuals. The body model is simply a tool designed to help you develop assessment skills by body area and navigate quickly though the simulation's learning activities. Review the diagram below to become familiar with the available Data Collection buttons and the additional options that appear when you click each button and body area.

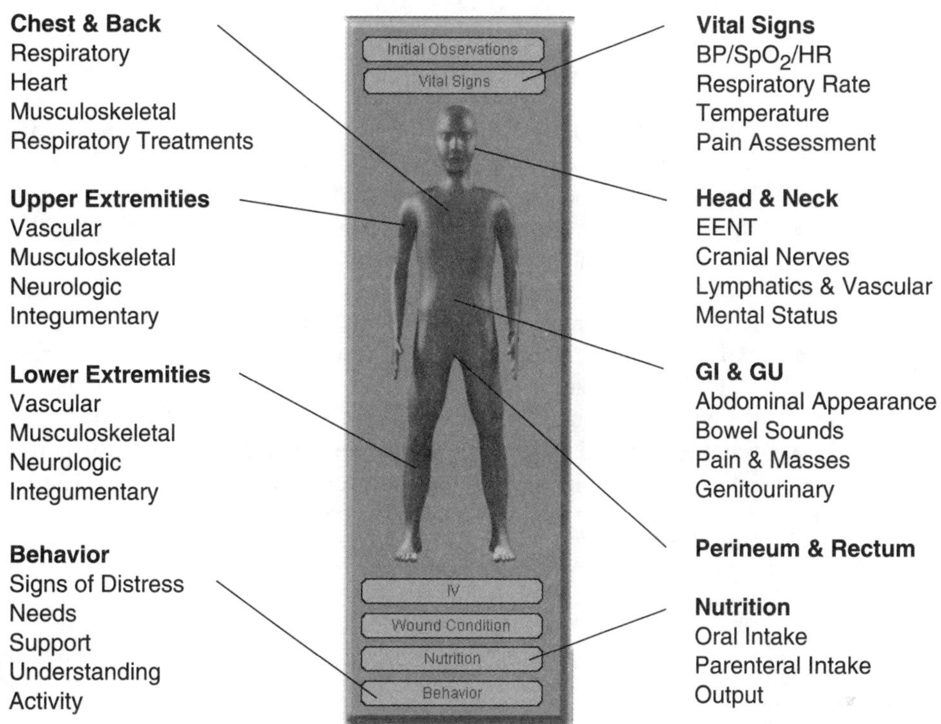

Whenever you click on an assessment button, either a video or still photo will be activated in the center of the screen. For some activities, data obtained during assessment are shown in a box to the right of that frame (see p. 14). For other assessment options, you must collect data yourself by observing the video—in these cases, no data appear in the box. You can always replay a video by simply reclicking the assessment button of the activity you wish to see again.

The *Virtual Clinical Excursions—Medical-Surgical* patient simulations were constructed by expert nurses to be as realistic as possible. As previously mentioned, the data for every patient will change through time. During the first 30 minutes of a period of care, you will generally find that all assessment options will give you data on the patient. However, after that period, some assessments may no longer be a high priority for a patient. The expert nurses who created the patient simulations let you know when an assessment area is not a high priority by sending you a short message. These messages appear in the box on the right side of the screen, where data are normally listed. Some examples of messages you might receive include "Please rethink your priorities for assessment of this patient" and "Your assessment should be focused on other areas at this time."

To leave the patient's room, click on the **Nurses' Station** button in the bottom right-hand corner of the screen. Note that this takes you back through the anteroom, where you must wash your hands before leaving. Once you have washed your hands, click on the outer door to return to the Nurses' Station.

Now, let's review what you just learned and try a few quick exercises to get a sense of how the Data Collection learning activities become available to you. You are already signed in to care for Elizabeth Washington, who was admitted following an auto accident in which her hip was fractured. Reenter her room from the Nurses' Station by clicking on **Patient Care** and then on **Data Collection**. You are now in the sink area of the patient's room, so wash your hands and click on the curtain to see the patient.

Start your patient care by collecting Ms. Washington's vital signs.

- Click on **Vital Signs**. Four assessment options will appear below the picture of the patient.
- Click on **BP/SpO$_2$/HR**. Watch the video as your preceptor measures blood pressure, oxygen saturation, and heart rate on a noninvasive multipurpose monitor. Record Ms. Washington's data for these attributes in the chart below.
- Now click on **Respiratory Rate**. This time, after a video plays, a "breathing" body model appears on the right. Measure Ms. Washington's respiratory rate by counting the respirations of the body model for the period of time your instructor recommends. Record your estimate of her respiratory rate below.
- Next, click on **Temperature**. First, you will see your preceptor measuring Ms. Washington's temperature; then the thermometer reading appears in the frame to the right. Record her temperature.
- Finally, assess Ms. Washington's pain by clicking on **Pain Assessment**. Note your interpretation of her pain. If she is in pain, record her pain level and characteristics.

Vital Signs	Time
Blood pressure	
SpO$_2$	
Heart rate	
Respiratory rate	
Temperature	
Pain rating	

Once you have collected Ms. Washington's vital signs, begin a lower extremities examination. Point your cursor to the leg area of the body model. Click anywhere on the orange highlighted area. Four new options now appear below the picture of your patient.

- Click on **Vascular**. Observe the video and review the data you obtain from this examination.
- Now click on **Neurologic**. Is Ms. Washington experiencing any numbness or tingling in her arms or legs?

You have now collected vital signs data and conducted a limited lower extremities assessment of Ms. Washington. As previously mentioned, most of the assessments combine a video or still photo of the patient with data that are collected for the respective assessment. Other assessments simply provide a video, and you must collect data from the nurse-patient interaction. For example, many of the pain assessments consist of the nurse asking the patient to rate his or her pain and the patient responding with a rating. Some of the behavior assessments also require that you listen to the nurse-patient interaction and make a decision about the patient's condition, needs, or psychosocial attributes.

When you visit patients in the Surgery Department, you will notice slightly different assessment options for some periods of care. However, the same types of interactions are always available. When you click on a button or area of the body model, you will be able to access a variety of patient assessments. If a video is shown, it can always be replayed by clicking on the assessment button.

HOW TO FIND AND ACCESS A PATIENT'S RECORDS

So far, you have visited a patient and practiced collecting data. Now you will examine the types of available patient records and learn how to access them. The records include the patient Charts, Medication Administration Record (MAR), Kardex plan of care, and Electronic Patient Record (EPR).

You are still signed in for Elizabeth Washington on the Medical-Surgical/Telemetry Floor, so let's explore her records. From the Nurses' Station, each type of patient record can be accessed in two ways. Practice both methods and choose the pathway you prefer. The first option is to use the menu in the upper left corner of the screen. First, click on **Patient Records**; this reveals a drop-down menu. Then select the type of patient record you wish to review by clicking on one of these options:

- **EPR**—Electronic Patient Record
- **Chart**—The patient's chart
- **Kardex**—A Kardex plan of care
- **MAR**—The current Medication Administration Record

You can also access patient records by clicking on various objects in the Nurses' Station. On the counter inside the station you will find a set of charts, a set of Kardex plans of care, a Medication Administration Record notebook, and a computer that houses the Electronic Patient Record system. All objects inside the Nurses' Station are labeled for quick recognition.

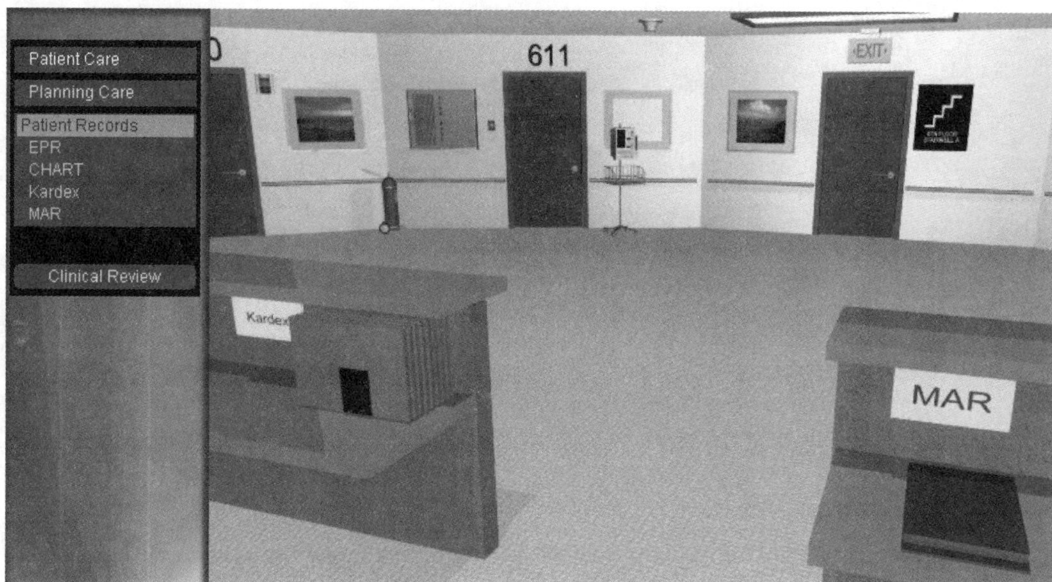

Chart

To open Ms. Washington's chart, click on **Chart** in the **Patient Records** drop-down menu—or click on the stack of Charts inside the Nurses' Station. Colored tabs at the bottom of the screen allow you to navigate through the following sections of the chart:

- History & Physical
- Nursing History
- Admissions Records
- Physician Orders
- Progress Notes
- Laboratory Reports
- X-Rays & Diagnostics
- Operative Reports
- Medication Records
- Consults
- Rehabilitation & Therapy
- Social Services
- Miscellaneous

To flip forward in the chart, select any available tab. Once you have moved beyond the first tab (History & Physical), a **Flip Back** icon appears just above the red cross in the lower right corner. Click on **Flip Back** to return to earlier sections of the chart. The data for each patient's chart are updated during a shift; updates occur at the start of a period of care. Note that some of the records in the chart are several pages long. You will need to scroll down to read all of the pages in some sections of the chart.

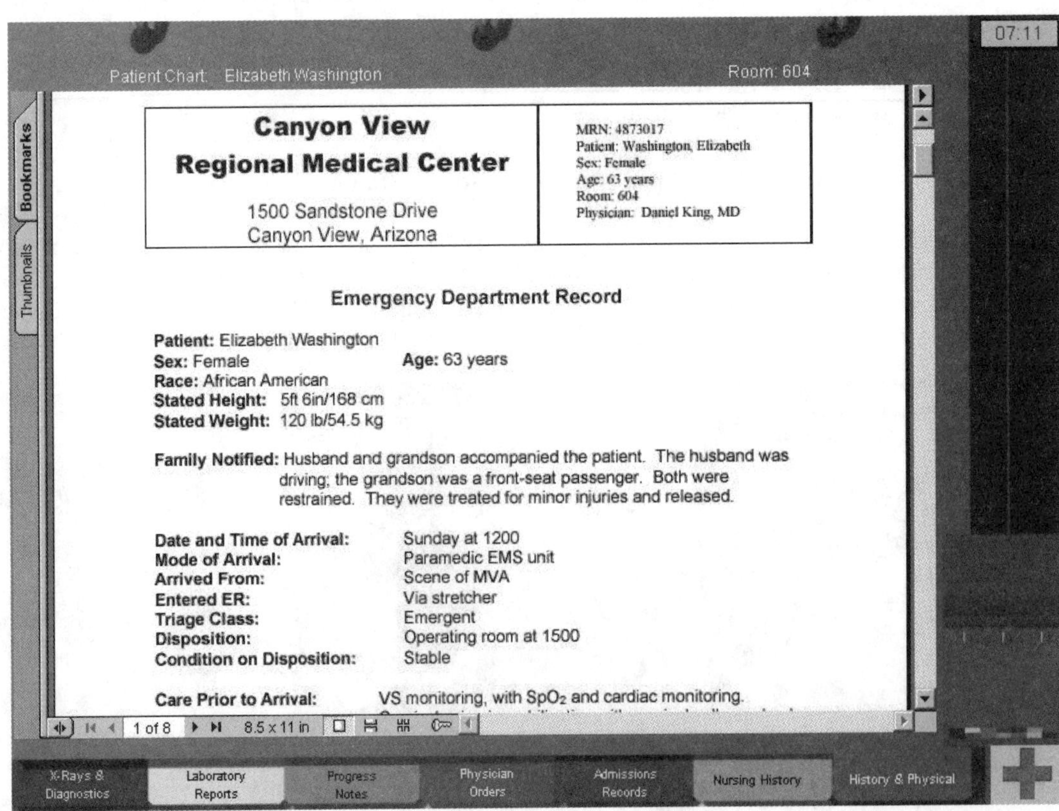

Canyon View Regional Medical Center
1500 Sandstone Drive
Canyon View, Arizona

MRN: 4873017
Patient: Washington, Elizabeth
Sex: Female
Age: 63 years
Room: 604
Physician: Daniel King, MD

Emergency Department Record

Patient: Elizabeth Washington
Sex: Female **Age:** 63 years
Race: African American
Stated Height: 5ft 6in/168 cm
Stated Weight: 120 lb/54.5 kg

Family Notified: Husband and grandson accompanied the patient. The husband was driving; the grandson was a front-seat passenger. Both were restrained. They were treated for minor injuries and released.

Date and Time of Arrival: Sunday at 1200
Mode of Arrival: Paramedic EMS unit
Arrived From: Scene of MVA
Entered ER: Via stretcher
Triage Class: Emergent
Disposition: Operating room at 1500
Condition on Disposition: Stable

Care Prior to Arrival: VS monitoring, with SpO_2 and cardiac monitoring.

Flipping forward and back through the various sections is accomplished by clicking on the tabs or on the **Flip Back** icon. To close a patient's chart, click on the **Nurses' Station** icon in the lower right corner of the screen.

Medication Administration Record (MAR)

The notebook under the MAR sign in the Nurses' Station contains the active Medication Administration Record for each patient. This record lists the current 24-hour medication orders for each patient. Double-click on the MAR to open it like a notebook. (*Remember:* You can also access the MAR through the Patient Records menu.) Once open, the MAR has tabs that allow you to select patients by room number. Each MAR lists the following information for every medication a patient is receiving:

- Medication name
- Route and dosage of medication
- Time to administer medication

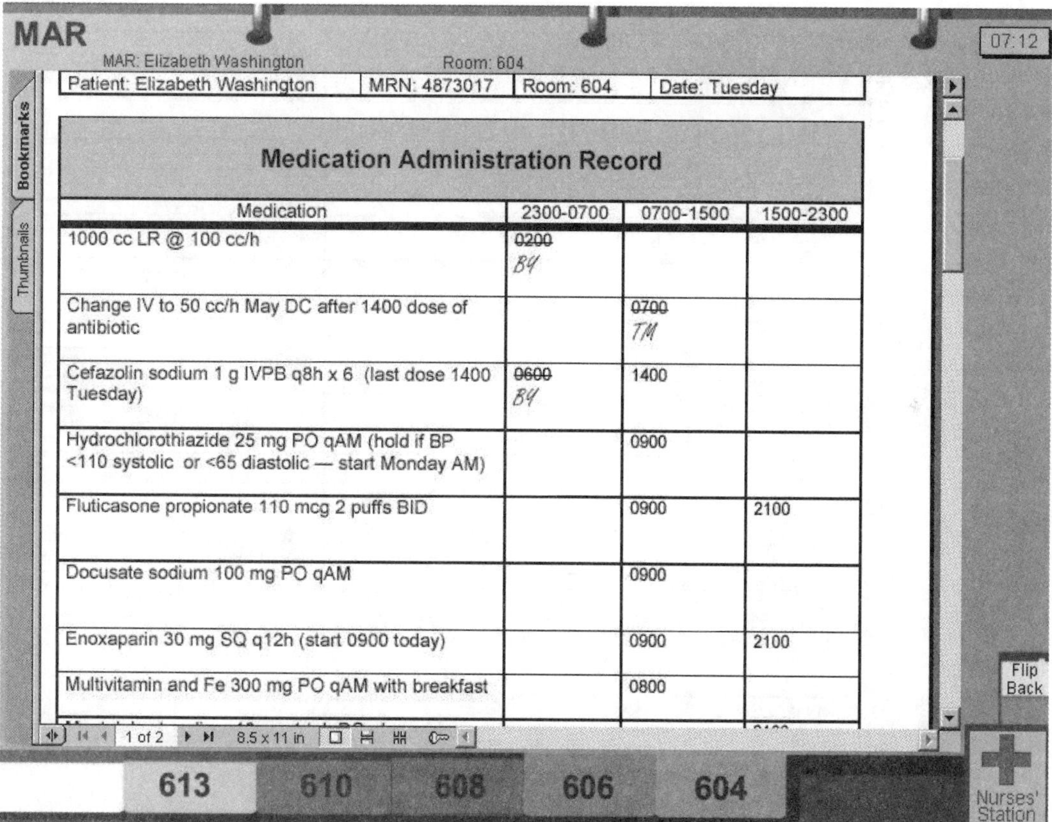

MAR

MAR: Elizabeth Washington Room: 604

Patient: Elizabeth Washington	MRN: 4873017	Room: 604	Date: Tuesday

Medication Administration Record

Medication	2300-0700	0700-1500	1500-2300
1000 cc LR @ 100 cc/h	~~0200~~ BY		
Change IV to 50 cc/h May DC after 1400 dose of antibiotic		~~0700~~ TM	
Cefazolin sodium 1 g IVPB q8h x 6 (last dose 1400 Tuesday)	~~0600~~ BY	1400	
Hydrochlorothiazide 25 mg PO qAM (hold if BP <110 systolic or <65 diastolic — start Monday AM)		0900	
Fluticasone propionate 110 mcg 2 puffs BID		0900	2100
Docusate sodium 100 mg PO qAM		0900	
Enoxaparin 30 mg SQ q12h (start 0900 today)		0900	2100
Multivitamin and Fe 300 mg PO qAM with breakfast		0800	

Scroll down to be sure you have read all the data. As with the patient charts, flip forward and back through the MAR by clicking on the patient room tabs or on the **Flip Back** icon. *Note:* Unlike the patient's Chart, which allows you to access data *only* for the patient for whom you are signed in, the MAR allows access to the data for *all* patients on the floor. Because the MAR is arranged numerically by patient room number, it is important that you remember to click on the correct tab for your current patient rather than reading the first record that appears on opening the MAR.

The MAR is updated at the start of every period of care. To close the MAR, click on the **Nurses' Station** icon in the lower right corner of the screen.

Kardex Plan of Care

Most hospitals keep a notebook in the Nurses' Station with each patient's plan of care. Canyon View Regional Medical Center's simplified plan of care is a three-page document modeled after the Kardex forms often used in hospitals. Access the Kardex through the drop-down menu (click **Patient Records**, then **Kardex**), or click on the folders beneath the Kardex sign in the Nurses' Station. *Note:* Like the MAR, the Kardex allows access to the plans of care for *all* patients on the floor. Side tabs allow you to select the patient's care plan by room number. Remember to click on the tab for your current patient rather than reading the first plan of care that appears after opening the Kardex. Scroll down to read all of the pages.

A Flip Back icon appears in the upper right corner once you have moved past the first patient's Kardex. Use the Nurses' Station icon in the bottom right corner to return to close the Kardex.

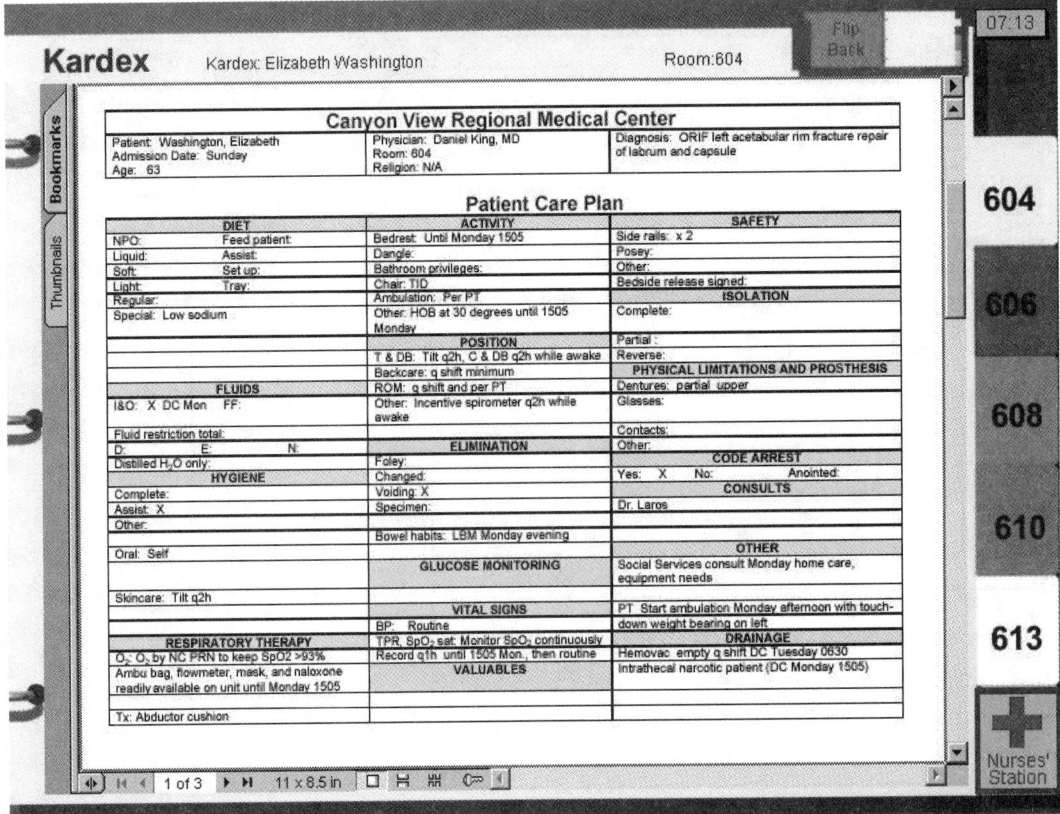

Canyon View Regional Medical Center

Patient: Washington, Elizabeth Admission Date: Sunday Age: 63	Physician: Daniel King, MD Room: 604 Religion: N/A	Diagnosis: ORIF left acetabular rim fracture repair of labrum and capsule

Patient Care Plan

DIET	ACTIVITY	SAFETY
NPO: Feed patient:	Bedrest: Until Monday 1505	Side rails: x 2
Liquid: Assist:	Dangle:	Posey:
Soft: Set up:	Bathroom privileges:	Other:
Light: Tray:	Chair: TID	Bedside release signed:
Regular:	Ambulation: Per PT	**ISOLATION**
Special: Low sodium	Other: HOB at 30 degrees until 1505 Monday	Complete:
	POSITION	Partial :
	T & DB: Tilt q2h, C & DB q2h while awake	Reverse:
	Backcare: q shift minimum	**PHYSICAL LIMITATIONS AND PROSTHESIS**
FLUIDS	ROM: q shift and per PT	Dentures: partial upper
I&O: X DC Mon FF:	Other: Incentive spirometer q2h while awake	Glasses:
Fluid restriction total:		Contacts:
D: E: N:	**ELIMINATION**	Other:
Distilled H_2O only:	Foley:	**CODE ARREST**
HYGIENE	Changed:	Yes: X No: Anointed:
Complete:	Voiding: X	**CONSULTS**
Assist: X	Specimen:	Dr. Laros
Other:		
	Bowel habits: LBM Monday evening	
Oral: Self		**OTHER**
	GLUCOSE MONITORING	Social Services consult Monday home care, equipment needs
Skincare: Tilt q2h		
	VITAL SIGNS	PT Start ambulation Monday afternoon with touch-
	BP: Routine	down weight bearing on left
RESPIRATORY THERAPY	TPR, SpO_2 sat: Monitor SpO_2 continuously	**DRAINAGE**
O_2: O_2 by NC PRN to keep SpO2 >93%	Record q1h until 1505 Mon., then routine	Hemovac empty q shift DC Tuesday 0630
Ambu bag, flowmeter, mask, and naloxone readily available on unit until Monday 1505	**VALUABLES**	Intrathecal narcotic patient (DC Monday 1505)
Tx: Abductor cushion		

Electronic Patient Record (EPR)

Some patient records are kept in a computerized system called the Electronic Patient Record (EPR). Although some hospitals have only limited electronic patient records—or none at all—most hospitals are moving toward computerized or electronic patient record systems.

The Canyon View EPR was designed to represent a composite of commercial versions used in existing hospitals and clinics. If you have already used an EPR in a hospital, you will recognize the basic features of all commercial or custom-designed EPRs. If you have not used an EPR, the Canyon View system will give you an introduction to a basic computerized record system.

You can use the EPR to review data already recorded for a patient—or to enter assessment data that you have collected. The EPR is continually updated. For example, when you begin working with a patient for the 11:00–12:29 period of care, you have access to all the data for that patient up to 11:00. The EPR contains all data collected on the patient from the moment he or she entered the hospital. The Canyon View EPR allows you to examine how data for different attributes have changed during the time the patient has been in the hospital. You may also examine data for all of a patient's attributes at a particular time. Remember, the Canyon View EPR is fully functional, as in a real hospital. Just as in real life, you can enter data during the period of care in which you are working, but you cannot change data from a previous period of care.

You can access the EPR once you have signed in for a patient. Use the Patient Records menu or find the computer in the Nurses' Station with **Electronic Patient Records** on the screen. To access a patient's EPR:

- Select the EPR option on the drop-down menu (click **Patient Records**, then **EPR**) or double-click on the EPR computer screen. This will open the access screen.
- Type in the password—this will always be **nurse2b**—but ***Do Not Hit Return*** after entering the password.
- Click on the **Access Records** button.
- If you make a mistake, simply delete the password, reenter it, and click **Access Records**.

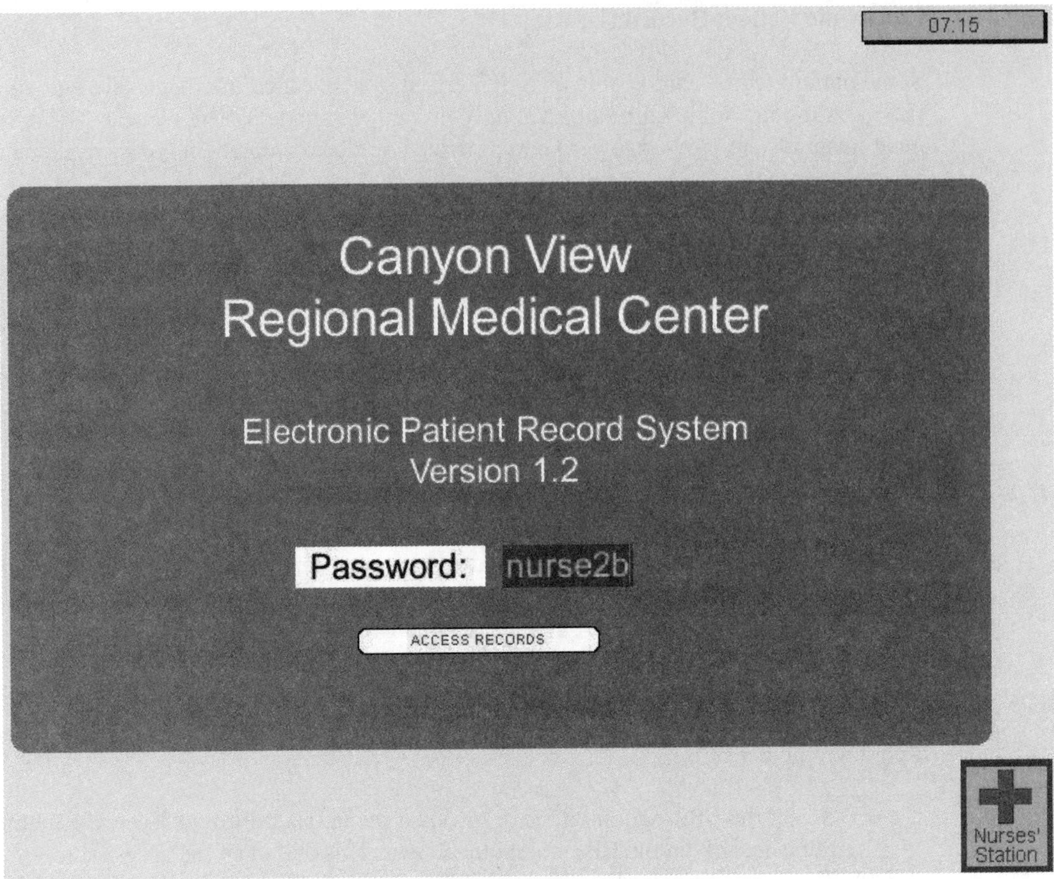

At the bottom of the EPR screen, you will see buttons for various types of patient data. Clicking on a button will bring up a field of attributes and the data for those attributes. You may notice that the data for some attributes appear as codes. The appropriate codes (and interpretations) for any attributes can be found in the code box on the far right side of the screen. Remember that every hospital or clinic selects its own codes. The codes used by Canyon View Regional Medical Center may be different from ones you have used or seen in clinical rotations. However, you will have to adjust to the various codes used by the clinical settings in which you work, so *Virtual Clinical Excursions—Medical-Surgical* gives you some practice using a system different from one you may already know. The different data fields available in the EPR are:

- Vital Signs
- Neurologic
- Musculoskeletal
- Respiratory
- Cardiovascular
- GI & GU
- IV
- Equipment
- Drains & Tubes
- Wounds & Dressings
- Hygiene
- Safety & Comfort
- Behavior & Activity
- Intake & Output

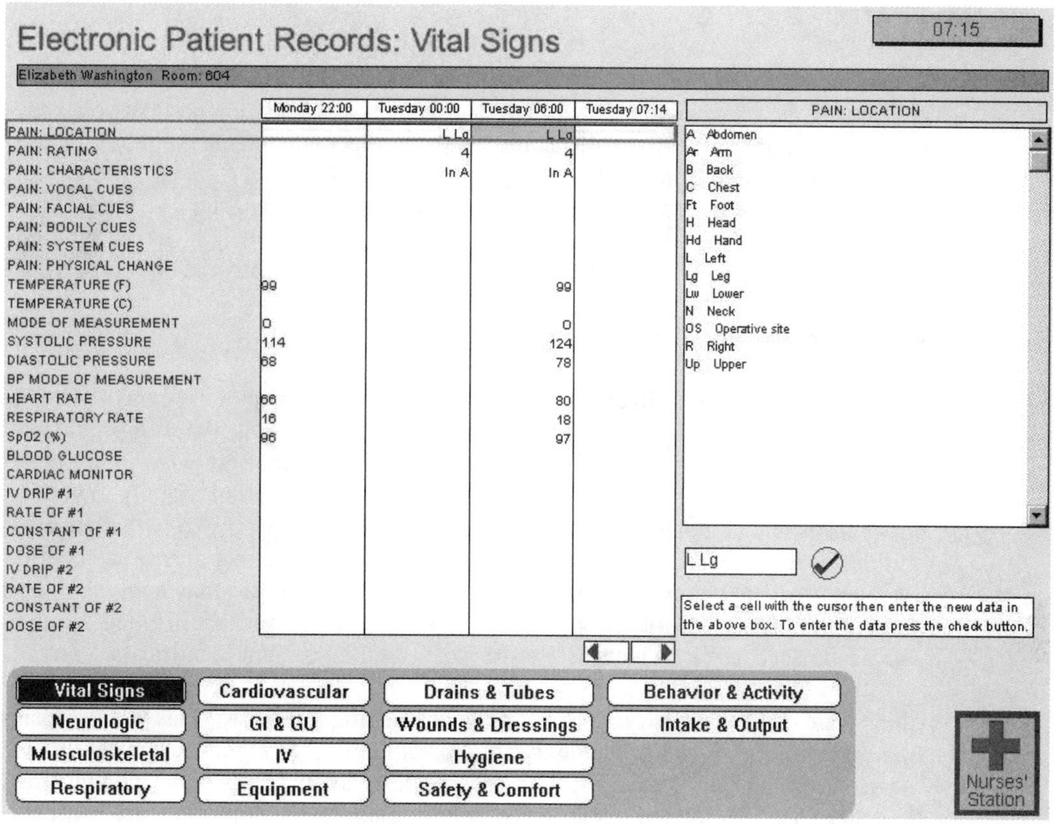

Electronic Patient Records: Vital Signs

07:15

Elizabeth Washington Room: 604

	Monday 22:00	Tuesday 00:00	Tuesday 06:00	Tuesday 07:14
PAIN: LOCATION		L Lg	L Lg	
PAIN: RATING		4	4	
PAIN: CHARACTERISTICS		In A	In A	
PAIN: VOCAL CUES				
PAIN: FACIAL CUES				
PAIN: BODILY CUES				
PAIN: SYSTEM CUES				
PAIN: PHYSICAL CHANGE				
TEMPERATURE (F)	99		99	
TEMPERATURE (C)				
MODE OF MEASUREMENT	O		O	
SYSTOLIC PRESSURE	114		124	
DIASTOLIC PRESSURE	68		78	
BP MODE OF MEASUREMENT				
HEART RATE	66		80	
RESPIRATORY RATE	16		18	
SpO2 (%)	96		97	
BLOOD GLUCOSE				
CARDIAC MONITOR				
IV DRIP #1				
RATE OF #1				
CONSTANT OF #1				
DOSE OF #1				
IV DRIP #2				
RATE OF #2				
CONSTANT OF #2				
DOSE OF #2				

PAIN: LOCATION

A Abdomen
Ar Arm
B Back
C Chest
Ft Foot
H Head
Hd Hand
L Left
Lg Leg
Lw Lower
N Neck
OS Operative site
R Right
Up Upper

L Lg

Select a cell with the cursor then enter the new data in the above box. To enter the data press the check button.

Vital Signs | Cardiovascular | Drains & Tubes | Behavior & Activity
Neurologic | GI & GU | Wounds & Dressings | Intake & Output
Musculoskeletal | IV | Hygiene
Respiratory | Equipment | Safety & Comfort

Nurses' Station

Click on **Vital Signs** and review the vital signs data for Elizabeth Washington. If you want to enter data you have collected for a particular attribute (such as pain characteristics), click on the data field in which the attribute is found. (Pain characteristics are found in the Vital Signs field.) Then click on the specific attribute line, and move the highlighted box to the current time cell. Blue arrows in the lower right corner move you left and right within the EPR data fields. Once the highlighted box is in the correct time cell, type in the code for your patient's pain characteristics in the box at the lower right side of the screen, just to the left of the check mark (√). Be sure to use the codes listed in the code box in the data entry area. Once you have typed the data in this box, click on the check mark (√) to enter and save them in the patient's record. The data will appear in the time cell for the attribute you have selected.

When you are ready to leave the EPR, click on the **Nurses' Station** icon in the bottom right corner of the screen.

PLANNING CARE

After assessing your patient, you must begin the careful process of deciding what diagnoses best describe his or her condition. For each diagnosis, you will list outcomes that you want your patient to achieve. Then, based on each outcome, you will select nursing interventions that you believe will help your patient achieve the outcomes you selected. *Virtual Clinical Excursions—Medical-Surgical* helps you in this process by providing a set of Planning Care resources. While you are still signed in for Elizabeth Washington, click on **Planning Care** in the upper left corner of the Nurses' Station screen. You will see two options: **Problem Identification** and **Setting Priorities**.

◆ Developing Nursing Diagnoses

Click on **Problem Identification**, and a note from your preceptor appears offering guidance about Ms. Washington's problems and possible diagnoses for the types of problems she may have. This diagnosis list is based on what expert nurses believe are *possible* for this particular patient. Remember, however, that not all of the diagnoses listed may apply to your patient—and that your patient may have other diagnoses that are not on the list. Your challenge and responsibility is to decide what nursing diagnoses *do* apply to your patient during each period of care. Since your patient's condition may be changing, some diagnoses may apply in one period of care but not in another. Read over the list of possible diagnoses for Elizabeth Washington. When you are finished, click on **Nurses' Station** to close the Problem Identification note.

Click again on **Planning Care**. This time select **Setting Priorities**. This will open another note from your preceptor. Notice that in the third paragraph of the note, your preceptor instructs you to use the Nursing Care Matrix. This is a resource designed to help you develop nursing diagnoses for your patient. To see how this resource works, click on the **Nursing Care Matrix** button at the bottom of the screen. Before you can develop nursing diagnoses, you must be sure your patient actually has the characteristics of those diagnoses. It is nearly impossible for anyone to remember all of the defining characteristics for every diagnosis, so nurses consult references such as *Nursing Diagnoses: Definitions and Classification, 2001–2002* (NANDA, 2001). To make your life a little simpler and to provide training in the health informatics resources of the future, the Nursing Care Matrix provides a list of diagnoses common for your type of patient, as well as the definition for each diagnosis and the defining characteristics for each diagnosis. Ackley and Ladwig (*Nursing Diagnosis Handbook: A Guide to Planning Care*, 5th edition) have mapped specific NANDA diagnoses onto major health-illness transitions. This mapping, along with input from our expert panel of nurses, provided the list of diagnoses you see—nursing diagnoses that *might* apply to Elizabeth Washington.

- Click on the first diagnosis. Note that the definition for this diagnosis now appears in a box in the upper right of the screen. The defining characteristics are listed in the box in the lower right of the screen.
- Click on another diagnosis. Review the definition and characteristics.

◆ Developing Outcomes and Interventions

For every nursing diagnosis you make, you can then select appropriate outcomes that you want your patient to achieve.

- Click on a diagnosis.
- Now click on **Outcomes and Interventions** at the bottom of the screen.
- On the left-hand side of the screen, you should now see the diagnosis you selected, along with a list of the outcomes you may want your patient to achieve if she has this diagnosis.

These outcomes are based on *Nursing Outcomes Classification*, 2nd edition (Johnson, Maas, and Moorhead, 2000). This reference provides detailed lists of linkages between the NANDA diagnoses and nursing outcomes defined in the *Nursing Outcomes Classification*.

For each outcome listed, you can access a list of nursing interventions to help your patient achieve that outcome.

- Click on the first outcome listed.
- On the right side of your screen, you will now see lists of intervention labels in three boxes: Major Interventions, Suggested Interventions, and Optional Interventions.

Each of the intervention labels in these boxes refers to an intervention that could be implemented to help achieve the specific outcome chosen. The *Nursing Intervention Classification* system gives a label to each intervention. Therefore, the Major, Suggested, and Optional Interventions are labels, each of which has a set of nursing activities that together comprise an intervention. If you look up a label in the *Nursing Interventions Classification*, you will see that it refers to a set of different nursing activities, some or all of which can be implemented in order to achieve the desired patient outcome for that diagnosis. We used *Nursing Diagnoses, Outcomes, and Interventions: NANDA, NOC and NIC Linkages* (Johnson, Bulechek, McCloskey-Dochterman, Mass, and Moorhead, 2001) and the *Nursing Interventions Classification*, 3rd edition, (McCloskey and Bulechek, 2000) to create the linkages between outcomes and interventions shown in the Nursing Care Matrix.

The Nursing Care Matrix provides you with a basic framework for learning how to move from making a diagnosis to defining patient outcomes and then to choosing the interventions you should implement to achieve those outcomes. Your instructor and the exercises in this workbook will help you develop this part of the nursing process and will provide you with more information about the nursing activities that belong with each intervention label.

CLINICAL REVIEW

Virtual Clinical Excursions—Medical-Surgical also incorporates a learning assessment system called the Clinical Review, which provides quizzes that evaluate your knowledge of your patient's condition and related conditions.

- If you are still in the Nursing Care Matrix, return to the Nurses' Station by clicking first on **Return to Diagnoses** at the bottom of the Outcomes and Interventions screen and then on **Return to Nurses' Station** at the bottom of the Diagnosis screen.
- From the menu options in the upper left corner, click on **Clinical Review**.
- You will now see a warning box that asks you to confirm that you wish to continue. Click **Clinical Review Center**.

You are now looking at the opening screen for the Clinical Review Center. You have three quiz options: **Safe Practice**, **Nursing Diagnoses**, and **Clinical Judgment**. Do not click on any quiz buttons yet. First, read the following descriptions of the quizzes you can select:

- **Safe Practice**
  The **Safe Practice** quiz presents you with NCLEX-RN–type questions based on the patient you worked with during this period of care. A set of five questions is randomly drawn from a pool of questions. Answer the questions, and the Clinical Review Center will score your performance.

- **Nursing Diagnoses**
  If you click on the **Nursing Diagnoses** button, you are presented with a list of 20 NANDA nursing diagnoses. You must select the five diagnoses in this list that most likely apply to your patient. The Clinical Review Center records your choices, gathers those choices that are correct, and scores your performance. The quiz then allows you to select nursing interventions for each of the outcomes associated with NANDA diagnoses that your correctly chose. For each of your correct diagnoses, you are presented with the likely outcomes for that diagnosis; for each outcome, you will see a list of six

nursing intervention labels. Only three of the intervention labels are appropriate for each outcome. You must select the correct labels. Again, your performance is automatically scored.

- **Clinical Judgment**
  The **Clinical Judgment** quiz asks you to consider a single question. This question evaluates your understanding of your patient's condition during the period of care in which you have just worked. Select your answer from four options related to your perception of your patient's stability and the frequency of monitoring you should be conducting.

You can take one, two, or all three of the quizzes. On any floor, when you are done with the quizzes, you must click on **Finish**. This will take you to a **Preceptor's Evaluation**, which offers a scorecard of your performance on the quizzes, discusses your understanding of the patient's condition and related conditions, and makes recommendations for you to improve your understanding.

Preceptor's Evaluation

	Clinical Review	
	Correct Responses	Score
Safe Practice	3.0	18.0
Implementing Nursing Care	4.0	16.0
Clinical Judgment	1.0	20.0
Totals		54.0
Total Score	Out of 100 possible points, you received 54.0 points or 54.0%	

Preceptor's Evaluation of Clinical Review

Clincial Judgment Recommendation - Congratulations! You made a good clinical decision about your client during this period of care

We want you to spend time practicing questions like those found in the Safe Practice assessment. These questions are very similar to those found on the NCLEX-RN. Also, we feel you need to study the nursing diagnoses approved by the North American Nursing Diagnosis Association (NANDA). Importantly, we want you to review the outcomes appropriate for a particular diagnosis as well as the interventions you would implement to achieve each outcome. You might want to spend time re-examining the diagnoses-outcomes-interventions linkages found in the Nursing Care Matrix. As mentioned above, the nursing diagnoses are based on approved diagnoses of the North American Nursing Diagnosis Association (NANDA). Remember that the outcomes are based on the Nursing Outcomes Classification and the interventions are based on the Nursing Interventions Classification (NIC).

Print a detailed report | Nurses' Station

Note: We don't recommend that you take any quizzes before working with a patient. The goal of *Virtual Clinical Excursions—Medical-Surgical* is to help you learn and prepare for practice as a professional nurse. Reading your textbook, using this workbook to complete the CD-ROM activities, and organizing your thoughts about your patient's condition will help you prepare for the quizzes. More important, this work will help you prepare for care of real-life patients in clinical settings.

HOW TO QUIT OR CHANGE PATIENTS

Eventually, you will want to take a short or long break, begin caring for a different patient, or exit the software.

◆ To Take a Short Break

- Go to the Nurses' Station.
- Click on **Leave the Floor**, an icon in the lower left corner of the screen.
- You will see a screen with a variety of options.
- Click on **Break** and you will be given a 10-minute break. This stops the clock. After 10 minutes you are automatically returned to the floor, where you reenter the simulation at the same moment in time that you left.

◆ To Change Patients

Choose option 1 or option 2 below, depending on which activities you have completed during this period of care.

1. Use the following instructions *if you have already completed one or more of the quizzes* in the Clinical Review Center for your current patient:

- Double-click on the **Supervisor's (Login) Computer** in the Nurses' Station.
- Read the instructions for logging in for a new patient and period of care.
- If you want to select a new patient on the *same* floor, click **Login**, select the new patient and period of care, and then click **Nurses' Station**.
- If you want to work with a patient on a *different* floor, click **Return to Nurses' Station**, take the elevator to the new floor, and sign in for the new patient on the Login computer in the Nurses' Station.

2. Use the following instructions *if you have* not *completed any of the quizzes* in the Clinical Review Center for your current patient:

- Double-click on the **Supervisor's (Login) Computer** in the Nurses' Station.
- Read the instructions in the Warning box. Then click on **Supervisor's Computer**.
- The computer logs you off and gives you the option of going to the Clinical Review Center or to the Nurses' Station. Unless you wish to go to the Clinical Review Center for evaluation of the period of care you just completed, click on **Nurses' Station**.
- Double-click on the **Login Computer** again, and follow the instructions to sign in for another patient. (See the third and fourth bullets in option 1 above for specific steps.)

When you visit the patients in the ICU (Floor 5), you will need to swap disks by following these steps:

- If up are currently signed in for a patient, go to the Supervisor's (Login) Computer and sign out. Return to the Nurses' Station.

- Leave the Nurses' Station and enter the elevator. Once you are inside the elevator, remove the disk from your CD-ROM drive and replace it with the other disk.

- Click on the button of the floor number where you need to go.

◆ To Quit the Software for a Long Break or to Reset a Simulation

- From the Nurses' Station, click on **Leave the Floor** in the lower left corner of the screen.
- You will see a new screen with a variety of options.
- You may select Quit with Bookmark or Quit with Reset.
  - **Quit with Bookmark** allows you to leave the simulation and return at the same virtual time you left. Any data you entered in the EPR will remain intact. Choose this option if you want to stop working for more than 10 minutes but wish to reenter the floor later at the exact point at which you left.
  - **Quit with Reset** allows you to quit and reset the simulation. This option erases any data you entered in the EPR during your current session. Choose this option if you know you will be starting a new simulation when you return.

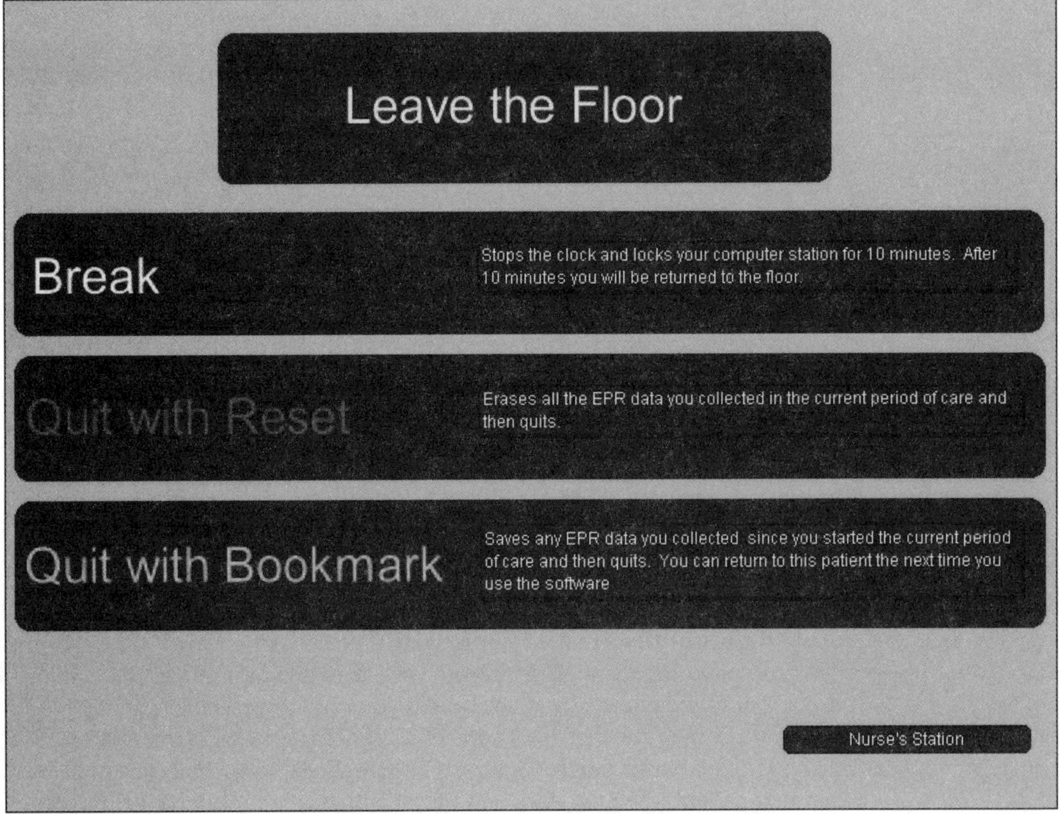

◆ To Practice Exiting the Software

- Click **Leave the Floor**.
- Now click **Quit with Reset**.
- A small message box will appear to confirm that you wish to quit and erase any data collected or recorded.
  - If you have reached this message in error, click the red X in the upper right corner to close this box. You may now choose one of the other options for leaving the floor (Break or Quit with Bookmark).
  - If you *do* wish to Quit with Reset, click **OK** on the message box.
- *Virtual Clinical Excursions—Medical-Surgical* will close, and you will be returned to your computer's desktop screen.

A DETAILED TOUR

What do you experience when you care for patients during a clinical rotation? Well, you may be assigned one or several patients that need your attention. You follow the nursing process, assessing your patients, diagnosing each patient's problems or areas of concern, planning their care and setting outcomes you hope they will achieve, implementing care based on the outcomes you have set, and then evaluating the outcomes of your care. It is important to remember that the nursing process is not a static, one-time series of steps. Instead, you loop through the process again and again, continually assessing your patient, reaffirming your earlier diagnoses and perhaps finding improvement in some areas and new problems in other areas, adjusting your plan of care, implementing care as planned or implementing a revised plan, and evaluating patient outcomes to decide whether your patients are achieving expected outcomes. Patient care is hands-on, action-packed, often complex, and sometimes frightening. You must be prepared and present—physically, intellectually, and emotionally.

Textbooks help you build a foundation of knowledge about patient care. Clinical rotations help you apply and extend that book-based learning to the real world. You will know this with certainty when you experience it yourself—for example, when you first read about starting an IV but then have to start an IV on an actual patient, or when you read about the adverse effects of a medication and you then observe these adverse effects emerging in a patient. Stepping from a book onto a hospital floor seems difficult and unsettling. *Virtual Clinical Excursions—Medical-Surgical* is designed as an intermediate tool to help you make the transition from book-based learning to the real world of patient care. The CD-ROM activities provide you with the practice necessary to make that transition by letting you apply your book-based knowledge to virtual patients in simulated settings and situations. Each simulation was developed by an expert nurse or nurse-physician team and is based on realistic patient problems, with a rich variety of data that can be collected during assessment of the patient.

Several types of patient records are available for you to access and analyze. This workbook, the software, and your textbook work together to allow you to move from ***book-based learning*** to real-life ***problem-based learning***. Your foundational knowledge is based on what you have learned from the textbook. The *VCE—Medical-Surgical* patient simulations allow you to explore this knowledge in the context of a virtual hospital with virtual patients. Questions stimulated by the software can be answered by consulting your textbook or reviewing a patient simulation. The workbook is similar to a map or guide, providing a means of connecting textbook content to the practice of skills, data collection, and data interpretation by leading you through a variety of relevant activities based on simulated patients' conditions.

To better understand how *Virtual Clinical Excursions—Medical-Surgical* can help you in your transition, take the following detailed tour, in which you visit three different patients.

■ WORKING WITH A MEDICAL-SURGICAL FLOOR PATIENT

In *Virtual Clinical Excursions—Medical-Surgical*, the Intensive Care Unit and Medical-Surgical/Telemetry Floor can be visited between 07:00 and 15:00, but you can care for only one patient at a time and only in the following blocks of time, which we call *periods of care*: 07:00–08:29, 09:00–10:29, 11:00–12:29, and 13:00–14:29. For each clinical simulation, you will select a single patient and a period of care. When you have completed the assigned care for that patient, you can then select a new patient and period of care. You can also reset a simulation at any point and work through the same period of care as many times as you want. Each time you sign in for a patient and time period, you will enter that session at the beginning of that period of care (unless you have previously "saved" a session by choosing Break or Quit with Bookmark).

Consider, for a moment, a typical Intesive Care Unit during the period between 07:00 and 15:00. Suppose that you could accompany a preceptor on that floor and provide care for patients during that 8-hour shift. Different expert nurses might take slightly different approaches, but almost certainly each nurse would establish priorities for patient care. These priorities would be based on report during shift change, a review of the patient records, and the nurse's own assessment of each patient.

At the beginning of a period of care, the assessment of each patient is usually accomplished by a general survey, that is, a fairly complete assessment of a patient's physical and psychosocial status. After the general survey, a nurse subsequently conducts focused assessments during the rest of the shift. The specific types of data collected in such focused assessments are determined by the nurse's interpretation of each patient's condition, needs, and applicable clinical pathways for independent and collaborative care. Depending on an agency's protocols and standards of care for the ICU patient, a nurse may conduct more than one comprehensive assessment during a shift, with focused surveys completed between the general surveys. Regardless of individual agency protocol, any ICU patient would have at least one general survey and numerous focused surveys over the period of the shift.

Now let's put these guidelines to practice by entering the ICU (Disk 1) at Canyon View Regional Medical Center. This time, you will care for James Story, a 42-year-old male suffering from renal failure.

1. Enter and Sign In for James Story

- Insert your *VCE—Medical-Surgical* Disk 1 in your CD-ROM drive and double-click on the **VCE—Medical-Surgical** icon on your desktop. Wait for the program to load.
- When Canyon View Regional Medical Center appears on your screen, click on the hospital entrance to enter the lobby.
- Click on the elevator. Once inside, click on the panel to the right of the door; then click on button **5** for the Intensive Care Unit (ICU).
- When the elevator opens onto the Intensive Care Unit, click on the **Nurses' Station**.
- Inside the Nurses' Station, double-click on the **Supervisor's (Login) Computer** and select James Story as your patient for the 09:00–10:29 period of care.

2. Case Overview

- Signing in automatically takes you to the patient's Case Overview. Your preceptor will appear and speak briefly on the video screen.
- Listen to the preceptor; then click on **Assignment** below the video screen.
- You will now see a Preceptor Note, which is a summary of care for James Story, covering the period of care just before the one you are now working.
- Review the summary of care. Scroll down to read the entire report.
- On the next page, make note of any information that you feel is important or that will require follow-up work, either with the patient or through examination of his records.

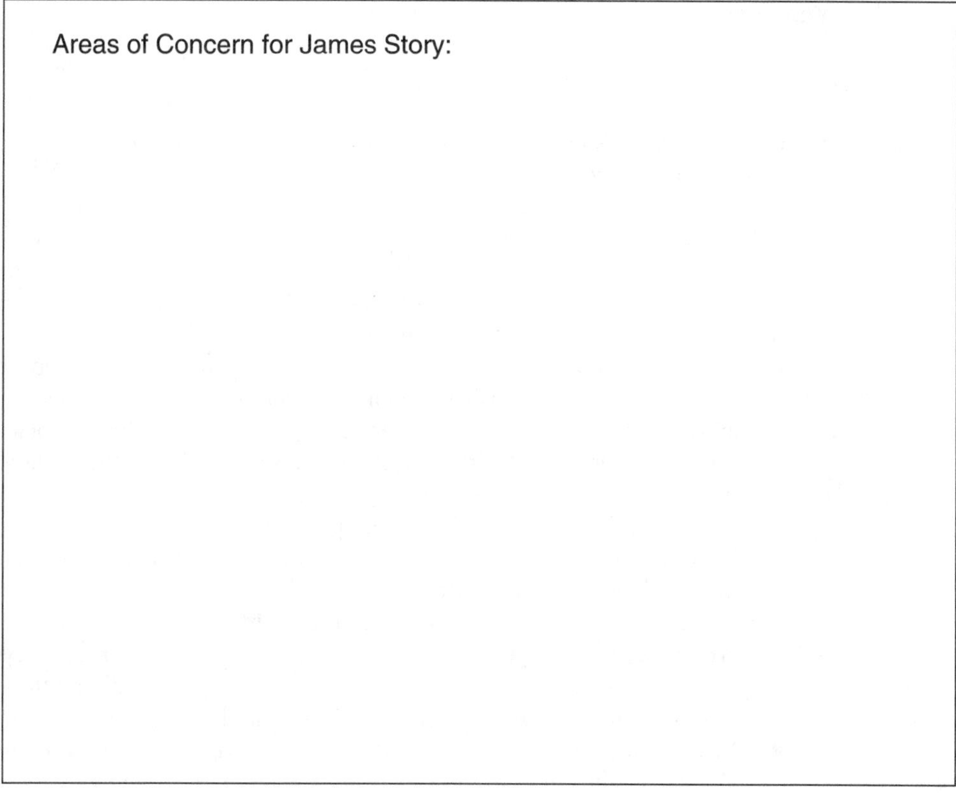

- When you have finished the case overview, click on **Nurses' Station** in the lower right corner of the screen and you will find yourself in the ICU Nurses' Station.

3. Initial Impressions

Visit your patient immediately to get an initial impression of his condition.

- On the menu in the upper left corner of your screen, click on **Patient Care**. From the options on the drop-down menu, click on **Data Collection**. *Remember:* You can also visit the patient by double-clicking on the door to his room (Room 512).
- In the anteroom, wash your hands by double-clicking on the sink. Then click on the curtain to enter the patient area.
- Inside the room, you will see many different options for assessing this patient. First, click on **Initial Observations** in the top left corner of the screen. Observe and listen to the interaction between the nurse preceptor and the patient. Note any areas of concern, issues, or assessments that you may want to pursue later.
- Now that you have gotten an initial impression of your patient, you have a few choices. In some cases, you might wish to leave the patient and access his records to develop a better understanding of his condition and what has happened since he was admitted. However, let's stay with Mr. Story a while longer to conduct a few physical and psychosocial assessments.

4. Vital Signs

Obtain a full set of vital signs from James Story.

- Click on **Vital Signs** (just below the Initial Observations button). This activates a pathway that allows you to measure all or just some of your patient's vital signs. Four options now appear under the picture of James Story. Clicking on any of these options will begin a data collection sequence (usually a short video) in which the respective vital sign is measured. The vital signs data change over time to reflect the temporal changes you would find in a patient such as Mr. Story. Try the various vital signs options to see what kinds of data are obtained.
  - First, click on **BP/SpO_2/HR**. Wait for the video to begin; then observe as the nurse preceptor uses a noninvasive monitor to measure Mr. Story's blood pressure, SpO_2, and heart rate. After the video stops, the preceptor's findings appear as digital readings on a monitor to the right of the video screen. Record these data in the chart below. If you want to replay the video, simply click again on **BP/SpO_2/HR**. *Note:* You can replay any video in this manner—as often as needed.
  - Now click on **Respiratory Rate**. This time, after the video plays, an image of a breathing body model appears on the right. Count the respirations for the amount of time recommended by your instructor. Record your measurement below.
  - Next, click on **Temperature**. Again, a video shows the nurse preceptor obtaining this vital sign, and the result is shown on a close-up of a digital thermometer on the right side of the screen. Record this finding in the chart below.
  - Finally, click on **Pain Assessment** and observe as the nurse preceptor asks Mr. Story about his pain. Note Mr. Story's response in the chart below.

Vital Signs	Time
Blood pressure	
SpO_2	
Heart rate	
Respiratory rate	
Temperature	
Pain rating	

5. **Mental Status**

From some of your vital signs assessments, you should be starting to form an idea of Mr. Story's mental status. However, you can check his mental status more specifically by doing the following:

- On the left side of the Data Collection screen is a body model. When you move your cursor along the body, it begins to rotate and the area beneath your cursor is highlighted in orange.
- Place your cursor on the head area of the body model and click.
- Notice that new assessment options now appear under the picture of your patient.
- Click on **Mental Status** (the bottom option of the list).
- Observe Mr. Story's responses and interactions with the nurse. Then review the data, if any, that appear to the right after the video has stopped.

6. **Respiratory Assessment**

Auscultate Mr. Story's lungs to see whether there is any evidence of adventitious lung sounds.

- Click on the chest area of the body model.
- Note the new assessment options that come up beneath the picture of Mr. Story.
- Click on **Respiratory**.
- Observe the examination of the anterior, lateral, and posterior chest. Then review the data collected by your preceptor.
- Do you believe there is any evidence of problems? If so, explain what data support your conclusion.
- If you were worried about potential problems, what other assessments might you conduct?

7. **Behavior**

Since this is your first visit with Mr. Story, you may also want to collect some psychosocial data.

- At the bottom left corner of the screen, click on **Behavior**.
- One at a time, click on each of the behavioral assessment options that appear below the picture of Mr. Story.
- As you observe each assessment, take notes on the nurse-patient interactions.
- Do any of his responses concern you?
- Does he have family support as well as nursing support?
- What other questions do you want to ask Mr. Story? When might you ask these questions?

8. **Chart**

You have conducted your preliminary examination of James Story. Next, review his patient records.

- To access the patient Charts, either click on the stack of charts inside the Nurses' Station or click on **Patient Records** and then **Chart** from the drop-down menu.
- James Story's Chart automatically appears since you are signed in to care for him. As described earlier in **A Quick Tour**, the Chart is divided into several sections. Each section is marked by a colored tab at the bottom of the screen. To flip forward and back through the Chart sections, click on the labeled tabs and on the **Flip Back** icon, respectively. Once you have moved beyond a section, the tab for that section disappears. You can move back to previous sections *only* by clicking on the **Flip Back** icon, which appears above the Nurses' Station icon in the lower right corner.

- Review the following sections of Mr. Story's chart: History & Physical, Nursing History, Operative Reports, and Progress Notes.
- Based on your analyses of these records and your preliminary assessment of Mr. Story, summarize key issues for this patient's care in the box below.
- When you are finished, close the chart by clicking on the **Nurses' Station** icon.

Key Issues for Patient Care:

9. Electronic Patient Record (EPR)

Now examine the data in James Story's EPR.

- To access the EPR, first click **Patient Records** in the upper left corner of the screen. Then click **EPR** on the drop-down menu. *Remember:* As an alternative, you can also double-click on the EPR computer in the Nurses' Station. This computer is located to the left of the Kardex and has **Electronic Patient Records** on the screen.
- On the EPR access screen, enter the password—**nurse2b**—and click **Access Records**.
- The EPR automatically opens to the patient's Vital Signs summary. Examine James Story's vital signs data for the past 8 hours.
- Now click **Respiratory** (three buttons below Vital Signs). The data from assessments of Mr. Story's respiratory system are now shown.
- Examine Mr. Story's data. Record your findings in the box on the next page.

Lung Sounds During the Past 24 Hours:

- Next, click on **Cardiovascular**.
- Review data collected for edema.
- List any evidence for fluid retention as evidenced by edema.
- If edema was observed, make sure you note the location(s) and quality.
- Note any other data that indicate problems.
- Now, make an assessment of Mr. Story's clinical status:

Cardiovascular Data:

a. Are any of the vital signs data you collected this morning significantly different from the baselines for those vital signs?

Circle One: Yes No

b. If "Yes," which data are different?

c. Do you have any concerns about the data collected during your respiratory assessment?

Circle One: Yes No

d. If you answered "No," what data tell you the patient is stable?

e. If you answered "Yes," what are your concerns?

10. Medication Administration Record (MAR)

- James Story has been taking a number of medications. Access his current MAR by double-clicking on the notebook below the MAR sign in the Nurse' Station. You can also open the MAR by clicking on **Patient Records** and then on **MAR** on the drop-down menu.
- Once the MAR notebook is open, access Mr. Story's records by clicking on the tab with his room number (512) at the bottom of the screen.
- Examine the MAR and note any medications that Mr. Story should be given during the period of care between 09:00 and 10:29. Make a list of these medications, the times they are to be administered, and any assessments you should conduct before and after giving the medications.

Medication Data:

- Click the **Nurses' Station** icon to close the MAR.

11. Planning Care

So far, you have completed a preliminary examination of James Story and reviewed some of his records. Now you can begin to plan his care. *Note:* Before *actually* starting a plan of care, you would conduct a more thorough assessment and a more complete review of this patient's records. However, let's continue so that you can learn how to use *Virtual Clinical Excursion's* unique and valuable Planning Care resource.

- On the drop-down menu, click **Planning Care** and then **Problem Identification**.
- Read the Preceptor Note for James Story and write one nursing diagnosis that you think might apply to this patient. Base your decision on your preliminary assessment and review of his records.

Nursing Diagnosis:

- Click on **Nurses' Station** to close this note.
- Click again on **Planning Care** in the upper left corner of your screen. This time, select **Setting Priorities** from the drop-down menu.
- Review the Preceptor Note on setting priorities for James Story.
- When you have finished, click on **Nursing Care Matrix** at the bottom of your screen.
- You will now see a list of nursing diagnoses approved by the North American Nursing Diagnosis Association (NANDA) that may apply to Mr. Story's condition.
- Find the diagnosis you just identified for Mr. Story. Click on this diagnosis.

- Review the nursing diagnosis definition and the defining characteristics that now appear on the right side of the screen.
- Does the definition fit your patient?
- Does your patient have the defining characteristics? If not, perhaps your assessment was not complete enough for you to make this decision. What other assessments should you conduct in order to determine whether this diagnosis applies to James Story?
- For now, assume that your diagnosis *does* apply to Mr. Story. Click on the **Outcomes and Interventions** button at the bottom of the screen.
- You now see a screen that lists nursing outcomes for your diagnosis. These are based on the Nursing Outcomes Classification. If your patient has this diagnosis, these are the outcomes you will want him to achieve.
- Some or all of these outcomes will probably apply to your patient if he does indeed have the nursing diagnosis you selected.
- Click on the first outcome, and text will appear in the three boxes on the right side of the screen. These boxes show the Major, Suggested, and Optional Interventions that could be implemented to achieve the outcome you selected, based on the Nursing Interventions Classification. *Remember:* Each entry listed in these boxes is an intervention label that represents a *set* of nursing activities that you would implement.
- Review the nursing interventions, especially those in the Major Interventions box. These are the most likely interventions you would implement to achieve the outcome you have clicked. However, you should consider all of the interventions before deciding which apply to the outcome for your patient.
- Now click on **Return to Diagnoses**. At this time, you can explore other diagnoses and their respective outcomes and interventions, or you can click **Return to Nurses' Station**.

Your work with James Story is completed for now. To quit the software and reset a simulation:

- Go to the Nurses' Station.
- Click on **Leave the Floor** in the lower left corner of the screen.
- A screen appears with a variety of options.
- Select **Quit with Reset**, which allows you to quit and reset the simulation. This option erases any data you entered in the EPR during your current session.

WORKING WITH A PERIOPERATIVE PATIENT

One of the patients at Canyon View Regional Medical Center, Darlene Martin, has been admitted to undergo a total abdominal hysterectomy.

- In the Surgery Department (Disk 2) on Floor 4, sign in to visit Darlene Martin for her Preoperative Interview.
- After viewing the Case Overview and reading the Assignment, return to the Nurses' Station. Click on **Patient Care** and then **Data Collection** on the drop-down menu.
- Wash your hands, enter the room, and click **View Interview**.
- After observing the interview, click on **Summary** and read the Preceptor Note.
- Now return to the Nurses' Station and sign out of this period of care.
- Click on the **Supervisor's (Login) Computer** again and sign in to visit Ms. Martin during her preoperative care.
- Although you cannot observe Ms. Martin's surgery, you can see her now in the Preoperative Care Bay and later in the PACU
- Once Ms. Martin is transferred out of PACU, you can visit her in her room on the Medical-Surgical/Telemetry Floor (Floor 6).

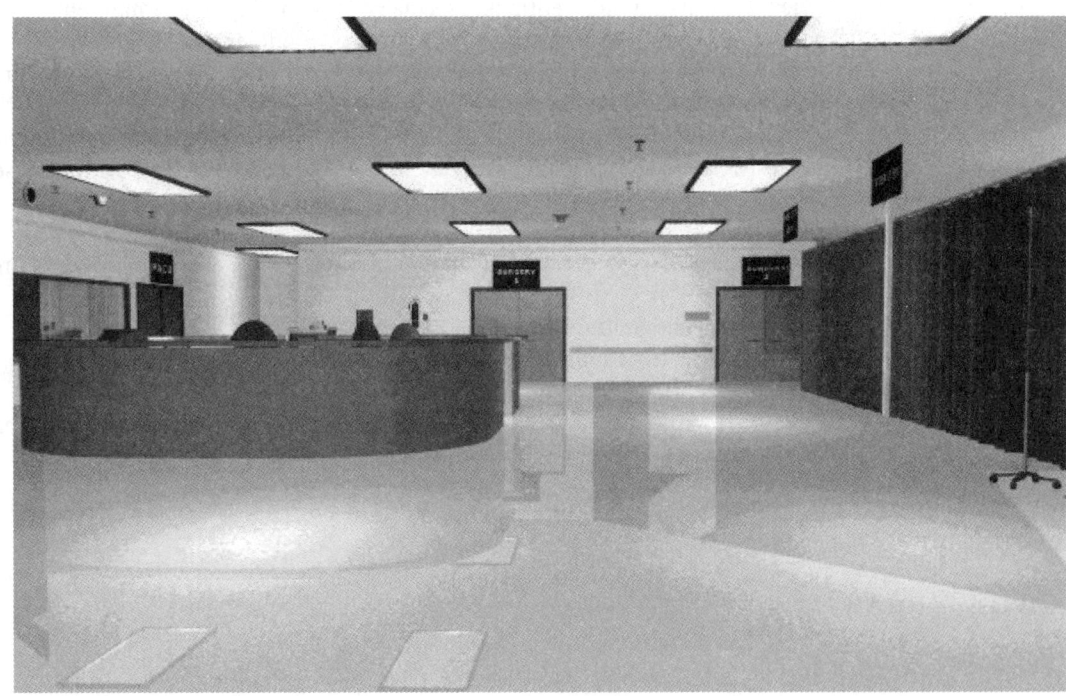

- Spend some time in each of the different perioperative settings in the Surgery Department, as described on p. 38. Then compare these perioperative settings with the settings on the Intensive Care Unit and the Medical-Surgical/Telemetry Floor. Use the following chart and focus your comparisons on the themes listed in the left column.

Comparison of Settings in Canyon View Regional Medical Center			
Activities and Resources	**Perioperative Settings**	**Intensive Care Unit Settings**	**Medical-Surgical/ Telemetry Floor Settings**
Patient Assessments			
Planning Care			
Types of Patient Records			

Remember: *Virtual Clinical Excursions—Medical-Surgical* is designed to provide a realistic learning environment. Within Canyon View Regional Medical Center, you will not necessarily find the same type of patient records, clinical settings, Nurses' Station layout, or hospital floor architecture that you find in your real-life clinical rotations. If you have already had experience within actual clinical settings, take a few moments to list the similarities and differences between the Canyon View virtual hospital and the real hospitals you have visited. There is considerable variation among hospitals in the United States, so think of *Virtual Clinical Excursions—Medical-Surgical* as simply one type of hospital and take advantage of the opportunity to practice learning how, where, when, and why to find the information, medication, and equipment resources you need to provide the highest quality patient care.

The following icons are used throughout the workbook to help you quickly identify particular activities and assignments:

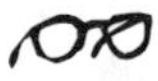 Indicates a reading assignment—tells you which textbook chapter(s) you should read before starting each lesson

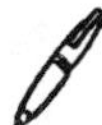 Indicates a writing activity

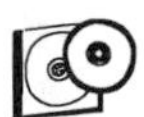 Marks the beginning of an interactive CD-ROM activity—signals you to open or return to your *Virtual Clinical Excursions—Medical-Surgical* CD-ROM

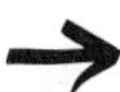 Indicates additional CD-ROM instructions

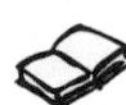 Indicates questions and activities that require you to consult your textbook

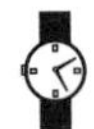 Indicates the approximate time required to complete an exercise

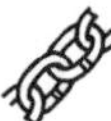 Indicates a link to another lesson

LESSON 1

Critical Thinking and Nursing Judgment

Reading Assignment: Critical Thinking in Nursing Practice (Chapter 14)
Nursing Assessment (Chapter 15)

Patients: James Story, Room 512
Julia Parker, Room 608

Objectives

- Identify how the nurse applies critical thinking to the assessment of a patient.
- Discuss the clinical decisions that apply in the case studies.
- Identify examples of critical thinking attitudes applied in the assessment of patients' health histories in the case studies.
- Describe how intellectual standards apply in patient assessment.
- Discuss ways in which reflection can improve a nurse's practice.
- Apply a critical thinking model to the care of patients in the case studies.

In every clinical situation, patients depend on nurses to be able to think critically and perform in a professionally competent manner. Critical thinking is essential to your ability to identify patient needs and to make the clinical decisions necessary for safe and appropriate care. Throughout any encounter with a patient, you must always use the skills of critical thinking: recalling past experiences that can help in the care of your current patient, reflecting on the knowledge that applies to a given patient's clinical condition, and anticipating and applying intellectual standards and critical thinking attitudes needed for a comprehensive approach to patient care.

Each patient poses a unique set of health care problems. Thus, when you first meet a patient, you will not always have a clear picture of the patient's needs and the appropriate nursing actions to take. Instead, you must learn to question, to wonder, and then to be self-directed in exploring the patient's condition and situation. Ultimately, the use of critical thinking will allow you to find a solution that can best help the patient.

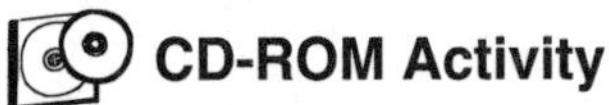

CD-ROM Activity

Exercise 1—James Story, Intensive Care Unit, Room 512

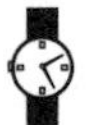

This exercise will take approximately 45 minutes to complete.

In this exercise you will visit James Story. He is a 42-year-old man who was admitted to the Emergency Department with symptoms of end-stage renal disease (ESRD).

- With *Virtual Clinical Excursions—Medical-Surgical* Disk 1 in your CD-ROM drive, click on the **Shortcut to VCE** icon on your desktop. (*Note:* See pp. 5–10 of the **Getting Started** section of this workbook for detailed instructions.)
- When the main entrance to Canyon View Regional Medical Center appears on your screen, click on the doors to gain entry.
- Click on the elevator; then click on the panel with the buttons for the various floors.
- When the close-up of the panel appears, click on button **5** to go to the Intensive Care Unit Floor (Floor 5).
- When the elevator doors open onto Floor 5, click on the central **Nurses' Station** to enter the station.
- Click and hold the mouse button while you move the mouse to the right or left until you see the Login Computer.
- Click on the **Login Computer** screen and follow the instructions for signing in.
- On the sign-in screen, select James Story as your patient and 07:00–08:29 as the period of care.
- Click on the **Nurses' Station** button in the lower right corner of the screen.
- A Case Overview screen will appear, and your preceptor will provide a brief report on your patient.
- Listen to the Case Overview on James Story.
- Click on the **Assignment** button to access the Summary of Report from your preceptor; focus on the patient history.

1. Complete the following form as you review the assignment history for Mr. Story.

Symptoms on admission:
Past medical history:
Sensory status:
Vital signs prior to surgery:

2. Match each of the following assessment data with the corresponding intellectual standard to indicate how the the history summary for Mr. Story could be more thorough.

	Intellectual Standard	Assessment Data
_____	Specific	a. Description of the extent of edema in leg
_____	Precise	b. Description of patient's perception of how visual problems affect his daily function
_____	Accurate	c. Description of time diarrhea began
_____	Significant	d. Measurement of the circumference of right arm

→ • Return to the Nurses' Station by clicking on the button in the bottom right corner of the screen.

- Click on **Patient Records** in the upper left side of the Nurses' Station screen and select **Chart** from the drop-down menu.
- Click on **Nursing History** and review.

3. An important part of critical thinking is to draw upon your knowledge base when assessing patient needs. As you review the Nursing History for James Story, what areas of knowledge do you believe are important to apply in order to assess his self-perception more thoroughly?

4. James Story's nursing history notes that the patient's "right arm is significantly edematous from shoulder to fingers." For each of the following intellectual standards, identify an assessment question/measurement you might use to better measure the extent of this clinical condition.

Complete

Relevant

Consistent

5. Match each assessment description with its type of data (subjective or objective).

	Assessment Description	Type of Data
_____	Bowel sounds hypoactive	a. Subjective data
_____	Patient states he feels terrible	b. Objective data
_____	Patient reports shortness of breath	
_____	Patient's weight is 174 pounds	
_____	Patient wears glasses	

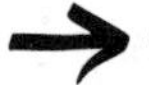

- Click on the **Nurses' Station** in the bottom corner of your screen to return there.
- Click on **Patient Care** and select **Data Collection** to go to Mr. Story's room.
- Wash your hands before you enter the room by first clicking in the sink and then on the faucet.
- Enter the room by clicking on the curtain on the right of the screen.
- Click on **Initial Observations** and observe the nurse conducting an assessment of Mr. Story.

6. Critical thinking involves a number of different competencies. Consider each of the scenarios below involving Mr. Story. Then describe the type of critical thinking competency that best describes each scenario.

   a. The nurse examines Mr. Story's dressing on the left hip and surrounding skin and notes moisture. The nurse palpates the dressing and finds it is dry. Then the nurse examines the connection of the infusion lock with the IV tubing and finds a leak at the connection site. The nurse changes the tubing.

   b. The nurse gathers information pertaining to Mr. Story's clinical status, including edema, weight, intake and output for 24 hours, and status of shortness of breath. The nurse determines the patient has a nursing diagnosis of Excess fluid volume.

   c. The nurse talks with Mr. Story about his concerns about dialysis and its effects on his lifestyle. He asks Mr. Story whether his wife can be included in the discussion. The nurse then talks with both individuals to determine the level of coping Mr. Story has shown and how they might work together to help him adapt to his disease.

7. Critical thinking is important in how you approach a problem or situation. Consider what you read in Mr. Story's Nursing History and then reflect on the information you observed during the data collection. Answer the following questions as they relate to Mr. Story.

   a. What needs to be achieved?

   b. What needs to be preserved?

   c. What needs to be avoided?

8. List, in order of importance, the priorities of nursing care you would set for Mr. Story.

9. Match each critical thinking attitude on the left with its description.

	Attitude	Description
_____	Fairness	a. The nurse decides to use several different nonpharmacologic approaches (guided imagery, relaxation) to relieve Mr. Story's pain and to improve his ability to sleep.
_____	Responsibility	b. The nurse decides to spend some time alone with Mr. Mr. Story's wife to learn as much as possible about how her caregiving for Mr. Story is affecting her own health.
_____	Perseverance	c. The nurse knows that he has difficulty caring for patients who do not adhere to therapy. He reflects on his concerns before talking with Mr. Story about his dialysis routine at home.
_____	Risk taking	d. The nurse has not cared for a patient with an AV graft before. Thus, he reviews the policy and procedure for dressing care of AV grafts.

CD-ROM Activity

Exercise 2—Julia Parker, Medical-Surgical Telemetry, Room 608

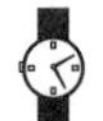

This exercise will take approximately 30 minutes to complete.

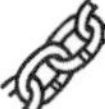

This exercise links to Lesson 15.

In this exercise you will visit Julia Parker, a retired psychologist who entered the ED with symptoms of indigestion and midback pain. She has experienced a myocardial infarction (heart attack). Ms. Parker is in the Medical-Surgical/Telemetry Unit on Floor 6, which can only be accessed from Disk 2. If you are just starting for the day and do not already have the software running, follow the first set of bulleted steps below. However, if you are continuing from Exercise 1 of this lesson, you do not have to quit and restart the program. Instead, follow the second set of bulleted steps below. (*Note:* Be sure you have Disk 2 nearby before you begin.)

If you are just starting the program for the day:

- With *Virtual Clinical Excursions—Medical-Surgical* Disk 2 in your CD-ROM drive, click on the **Shortcut to VCE** icon on your desktop. (*Note:* See pp. 5–10 of the **Getting Started** section of this workbook for detailed instructions.)
- When the main entrance to Canyon View Regional Medical Center appears on your screen, click on the doors to gain entry. Once inside the lobby, click on the elevator. From inside the elevator, click on the panel with the buttons for the various floors. When the close-up of the panel appears, click on button **6** to go to the Medical-Surgical Telemetry Unit (Floor 6).
- When the elevator doors open onto Floor 6, click on the central **Nurses' Station.**
- Click and hold the mouse button while you move the mouse to the right or left until you see the Login Computer.
- Click on the **Login Computer** screen and sign in to care for Julia Parker at 07:00–08:29.
- Click on the **Nurses' Station** button in the lower right corner of the screen.
- A Case Overview screen will appear, and your preceptor will provide a brief report on your patient. Listen carefully to the report on Ms. Parker.
- After listening to the report, proceed to the first arrow on the top of the next page.

If you are continuing directly from Exercise 1 of this lesson:

- First, you must log out from your current patient and period of care. To do so, click on the **Login Computer** screen, select the **Supervisor's Computer** button, and then click **Nurses' Station**. This logs you out and returns you to the 5th Floor Nurses' Station.
- Now, click and hold your mouse button and move your mouse to the left until you see the open elevator. Click inside the elevator to enter it.
- Once inside the elevator, double-click on the panel of floor buttons to the right of the open door. Then click on the button for **Floor 6**.
- The door of your CD-ROM drive should open automatically and your screen will prompt you to switch disks.
- Remove Disk 1 and insert *Virtual Clinical Excursions—Medical-Surgical* Disk 2 in the CD-ROM drive.
- Close the door to your CD-ROM drive and click again on button **6**.
- When the elevator doors reopen onto Floor 6, click on the **Nurses' Station** to enter the floor.
- Find and access the **Login Computer** and sign in for Ms. Parker at 07:00–08:29.
- Listen carefully to the Case Overview report.
- After listening to the report, proceed to the first arrow on the top of the next page.

→ Now that you have signed in to care for Ms. Parker and listened to her Case Overview, it's time to review her Chart and visit her in her room.

- Click on the **Nurses' Station** button in the bottom right corner of the screen to return there.
- Click on **Patient Records** on the left side of the screen and select **Chart**.
- Click on **Nursing History** and review.
- Return to the Nurses' Station and click on **Patient Care**. Select **Data Collection** to go to Julia Parker's room.
- Wash your hands by clicking in the sink and then on the faucet.
- Enter her room by clicking to the right of the sink.
- Click on **Behavior** on the lower left side of the screen.
- Click on each item on the menu that appears in the center of the screen and observe the nurse and patient interaction.

1. The nurse assessed Ms. Parker's signs of distress. During the patient and nurse interaction there were three communication strategies used by the nurse. List the three strategies. (*Hint:* Review interview techniques in textbook Chapter 15; also review Chapter 23 on Communication).

2. Ms. Parker has experienced losses and now is fearful of her future. Critical thinking applied to assessment enables a nurse to develop a relevant and comprehensive plan of care. Complete the following critical thinking diagram for assessment of Ms. Parker's situation by writing the letter of each critical thinking factor (listed on the next page) under its proper category below.

Knowledge

(1) ____________

(2) ____________

(3) ____________

Experience	**Assessment Julia Parker**	**Standards**
(4) ____________		(6) ____________
(5) ____________		(7) ____________
		(8) ____________

Attitudes

(9) ____________

(10) ____________

Critical Thinking Factors

a. Consider the time you had a personal loss and how it made you feel.
b. Review the long-term physiologic effects a myocardial infarction has on a patient's well-being.
c. Explore the meaning of Ms. Parker's loss of her husband and how that affects her perception of her ability to cope with her illness.
d. Review the theories of loss and grief.
e. Because Ms. Parker is a psychologist, ask her to describe what she would tell a patient who has experienced a loss and how she might relate personally to that advice.
f. Consider the therapeutic communication principles to use in building a trusting relationship with Ms. Parker.
g. Apply what you learned from caring for a patient newly diagnosed with a stroke to Ms. Parker's case.
h. Ask Ms. Parker to share in detail what fears she has about her heart attack.
i. Show your knowledge of Ms. Parker's situation by providing accurate information when she asks questions.
j. Ms. Parker stated in the nursing history that she did not know whether she could once again play with her grandchildren. Have her explain what she normally does when playing with the children.

3. Match each description with its corresponding phase of an interview.

	Description	Interview Phase
_____	Nurse summarizes important points discussed during the interview.	a. Orientation phase
_____	Nurse uses various techniques to gather information about patient's health status.	b. Working phase
_____	Nurse explains when there will be contact again with the patient in the future.	c. Termination phase
_____	Nurse explains to patient why data are collected.	
_____	Nurse uses communication strategies to focus on specific nature of patient's problems.	
_____	Nurse introduces self to patient.	

4. When using reflection in practice, a nurse purposefully thinks back or recalls the experience she or he had in caring for a patient. After observing the nurse's assessment of Ms. Parker's behavior, reflect on the nurse's performance. Is there anything you might have done differently if you had been the nurse?

LESSON 2

Applying the Nursing Process

Reading Assignment: Nursing Assessment (Chapter 15)
Nursing Diagnosis (Chapter 16)
Planning Nursing Care (Chapter 17)
Implementing Nursing Care (Chapter 18)
Evaluation (Chapter 19)

Patient: Paul Jungerson, Room 602

Objectives

- Assess the health care needs of patients in the case studies.
- Form data clusters from information gathered in nursing assessment.
- Develop nursing diagnoses from data presented in the case studies.
- Develop a concept map.
- Apply critical thinking to the nursing diagnostic process.
- Identify priorities of nursing care for a case study patient.
- Develop outcome statements.
- Develop a nursing care plan.
- Identify types of nursing interventions.
- Select evaluation methods appropriate to a patient's plan of care.

As a nurse, you will routinely apply the nursing process in your care of patients. Whether you care for a patient who suffers a life-threatening illness or you are counseling a mother with a new baby, the nursing process becomes your "set of tools" for ensuring that you know your patients' needs, select the right nursing therapies, administer your care, and evaluate its effectiveness. At first you will find yourself thinking very logically and systematically as you apply the nursing process in the care of patients. Each step of the process is a methodical and orderly approach to critical thinking. Eventually, as you acquire more experience, the nursing process becomes an automatic way of thinking critically and acting as a competent professional.

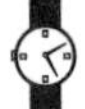

CD-ROM Activity

Exercise 1—Paul Jungerson, Medical-Surgical Telemetry, Room 602

This exercise will take approximately xx minutes to complete.

In this exercise you will visit Paul Jungerson. He is a retired postal worker who entered the hospital following a 3-day history of left lower quadrant pain. He had surgery Saturday for repair of a coloanal anastomosis with creation of a diverting transverse colostomy. You may have worked with Mr. Jungerson previously.

- With *Virtual Clinical Excursions—Medical-Surgical* Disk 2 in your CD-ROM drive, click on the **Shortcut to VCE** icon, enter the hospital, and take the elevator to Floor 6. (*Note:* If you need help with these steps, see pp. 5–10 of the **Getting Started** section of this workbook.)
- Click on the central **Nurses' Station**.
- Find and click on the **Login Computer**.
- Log in to visit Paul Jungerson during the time 07:00–08:29.
- Click on the **Nurses' Station** button in the lower right corner of the screen.
- Listen to the Case Overview; then click on **Assignment** and read the Preceptor Note.
- Click on the **Nurses' Station** button in the bottom right corner of the screen.

1. Reviewing the Case Overview and Assignment is similar to receiving an end-of-shift report. As the nurse assuming care for Mr. Jungerson, it is important for you to establish a database for your shift of care. Based on what you know from the Assignment, identify six potential problem areas to assess for Mr. Jungerson.

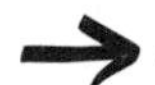

- Click on **Patient Care** and select **Data Collection** from the drop-down menu.
- Wash your hands by first clicking in the sink and then on the faucet.
- Enter Mr. Jungerson's room by clicking on the curtain on the right of the screen.
- Click on the buttons on the left of your screen and view the nurse's assessment for each of the six problem areas you identified in question 1.

2. Fill out the data sheet below as you observe the nurse's assessment of Mr. Jungerson.

Vital signs
Comfort level
Respiratory
Wound
Elimination/ostomy
IV

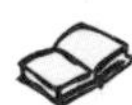

3. Assessment data must be descriptive, concise, and complete. The nurse asked Mr. Jungerson whether his pain was in the same area and whether there was radiation. List three additional questions that the nurse might have asked. (*Study Tip:* Review pain assessment in Chapter 42 of your textbook.)

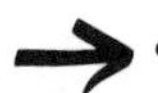

- Click on **Nurses' Station**.
- Select **Patient Records** and click on **Chart**.
- Click on **Nursing History** and read this section of Mr. Jungerson's Chart.

4. Data can be subjective or objective information. Match each of the following examples of assessment data with its corresponding data type.

	Assessment Data	Data Type
_____	Says "Keep me informed; teach me about this colostomy care."	a. Subjective Data
		b. Objective Data
_____	Reports fear of surgery and living with cancer	
_____	Frequently awake during the night	
_____	When asked about quality of sleep, says it is "OK"	
_____	Prefers demonstration and reading for instruction	

5. After gathering assessment data, it is important for the nurse to validate the information. How might the nurse validate data pertaining to Mr. Jungerson?

6. There is enough information in Mr. Jungerson's nursing history to form clusters of data. Organize the data listed below into three clusters.

Cluster I ___________

Cluster II ___________

Cluster III ___________

a. Fatigued because of sleeplessness

b. Anxious about living with colostomy

c. Drinks beer before going to bed

d. Wife died in 1999

e. Says "Keep me informed about colostomy"

f. Describes stress from change in lifestyle

g. Frequently awake during night

h. Prefers demonstration and reading

i. Son lives in Akron

j. Has problem getting to sleep

k. Has decreased eye contact when he discusses wife

7. The nursing diagnostic process requires analysis and interpretation of data. Let's take one cluster of data identified for Mr. Jungerson. Review the data listed in the first box; then fill in the other two boxes below.

Data Clustering

Fatigued because of sleeplessness
Drinks beer before going to bed
Frequently awake during night
Has problem getting to sleep

Defining Characteristics

Patient Need

8. When focusing on patterns of data, compare Mr. Jungerson's pattern with data that are consistent with normal, healthful patterns. What norms might you apply to your sleep data in question 7?

9. Formulation of a nursing diagnosis should be accurate to ensure that appropriate and relevant therapies are eventually chosen for a patient. Identify the diagnostic label that best describes the essence of Mr. Jungerson's response to health conditions.

10. The related factor of a diagnosis is the condition(s) influencing the patient's response to the health problem—in this case, Mr. Jungerson's disturbed sleep. For each of the related factors below, explain what the focus of nursing intervention would be.

Related Factors	Focus of Nursing Intervention
Biochemical agents (e.g., caffeine, alcohol)	
Anxiety	
Grief	

- Before selecting a related factor for Mr. Jungerson's diagnosis of Disturbed sleep pattern, you might want more data. Return to the Nurses' Station.
- Select **Patient Care** and click on **Data Collection**. (Remember to wash your hands before entering the patient's room.)
- Click on the **Behavior** button and review the behavior assessment for Mr. Jungerson.

11. The nursing diagnosis of Disturbed sleep pattern related to grief is an example of a:
    a. wellness nursing diagnosis.
    b. risk nursing diagnosis.
    c. actual nursing diagnosis.
    d. potential nursing diagnosis.

12. Which of the following examples is a correctly worded diagnostic statement?
    a. Dysfunctional grieving related to inability to accept loss of wife.
    b. Continued grieving related to inability to accept loss.
    c. Patient needs to resolve grief related to loss of wife.
    d. Provide frequent support because of dysfunctional grief response.

CD-ROM Activity

Exercise 2—Paul Jungerson, Medical-Surgical Telemetry, Room 602

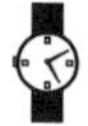

This exercise will take approximately 30 minutes to complete.

In this exercise you will visit Paul Jungerson, a retired postal worker who entered the hospital following a 3-day history of left lower quadrant pain. He had surgery Saturday for repair of a coloanal anastomosis with creation of a diverting transverse colostomy. You may have worked with Mr. Jungerson previously.

- With *Virtual Clinical Excursions*—Medical-Surgical Disk 2 in your CD-ROM drive, click on the **Shortcut to VCE** icon, enter the hospital, and take the elevator to Floor 6.
- Click on the central **Nurses' Station**.
- Find and click on the **Login Computer**.
- Log in to visit Paul Jungerson during the time 13:00–14:29.
- Listen to the Case Overview; then click on **Assignment** and review the Preceptor Note.
- Click on **Nurses' Station**.
- Click on **Patient Care** and select **Data Collection** from the drop-down menu.
- Wash your hands by first clicking in the sink and then on the faucet.
- Enter the room by clicking on the curtain on the right of the screen.
- Review the nurse's assessments in the following categories: **Initial Observations, Vital Signs** (specifically **Pain Assessment**), **GI & GU,** and **Behavior.**

1. Mr. Jungerson's condition is changing. On the basis of information gathered from the nurse's assessment, in addition to information from Exercise 1, Mr. Jungerson has a number of health needs and problems. For each of the following health needs or problems, identify the level of priority.

	Health Need/Problem	**Level of Priority**
_____	Grief	a. High priority
_____	Sleep	b. Intermediate priority
_____	Deficient knowledge	c. Low priority
_____	Acute pain	
_____	Paralytic ileus	

2. Planning for Mr. Jungerson's care will require the application of critical thinking. There are many factors to consider in how to assist Mr. Jungerson toward recovery. Complete the following critical thinking diagram for planning Mr. Jungerson's care.

Knowledge

(1) ___________

(2) ___________

(3) ___________

Experience

(4) ___________

Assessment
Paul Jungerson

Standards

(5) ___________

(6) ___________

(7) ___________

Attitudes

(8) ___________

(9) ___________

Critical Thinking Factors

a. Consider Mr. Jungerson's surgical report describing colon resection.
b. Use the same pain scale each time you assess Mr. Jungerson's discomfort.
c. Apply teaching/learning principles to select appropriate teaching methods.
d. Admit what you do not know about ostomy care and seek assistance from an ostomy therapist as needed.
e. Reflect on what you have learned in caring for previous abdominal surgical patients.
f. Show confidence as you work with Mr. Jungerson in planning pain management therapies.
g. Review principles of the grief response and the influence on physical well-being.
h. Follow the ethical standard of autonomy in supporting decisions made by Mr. Jungerson about his care.
i. Include in your teaching plan information relevant to Mr. Jungerson's lifestyle so that he can easily manage his colostomy.

3. When planning care, you establish goals and expected outcomes for each nursing diagnosis. Listed below are four different nursing diagnoses, along with a list of goals and outcomes. For each nursing diagnosis, choose an appropriate goal and outcome.

Nursing Diagnoses

Acute pain:

Goal _____

Outcome _____

Dysfunctional grieving:

Goal _____

Outcome _____

Disturbed sleep pattern:

Goal _____

Outcome _____

Deficient knowledge:

Goal _____

Outcome _____

Goals

a. Patient will perform ostomy self-care.

b. Patient will obtain sense of restfulness following sleep.

c. Patient will establish new relationships.

d. Patient will achieve pain relief.

Outcomes

e. Patient will have fewer than two awakenings during the night.

f. Patient will report pain as 2 or lower on scale of 0 to 10.

g. Patient will demonstrate ostomy pouch change.

h. Patient will discuss feelings about loss of wife.

4. There are seven different guidelines for writing goals and expected outcomes. List four of those guidelines.

5. Explain what is inaccurate in each of the following goal/outcome statements.

   a. Patient will achieve a minimum of 7 to 8 hours of sleep and fall asleep within 30 minutes by 4/22.

   b. Patient will identify signs to report indicating stomal dysfunction.

c. Patient will achieve normal sleep within 2 weeks.

d. Instruct patient on skin care measures by 4/24.

6. Mr. Jungerson has been identified as having the following nursing diagnoses: Disturbed sleep pattern, Acute pain, and Dysfunctional grief. On the concept map below, draw lines with arrows to show which diagnoses are interrelated.

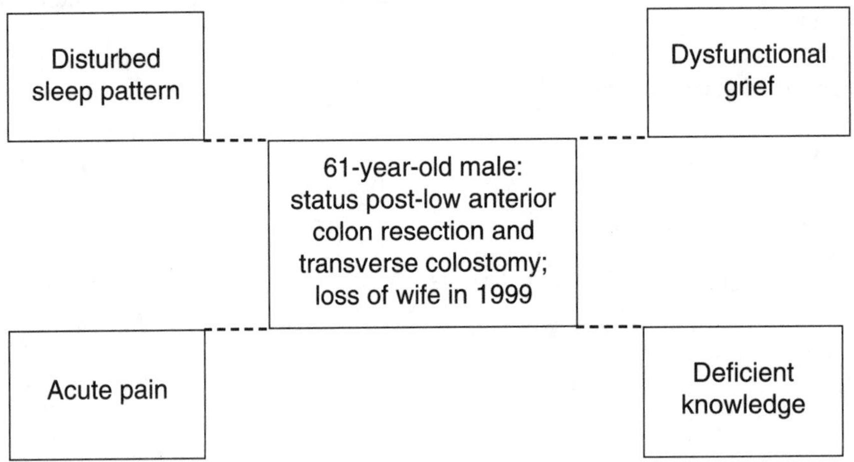

7. Mr. Jungerson will require a number of interventions in his plan of care. For each of the interventions listed below, identify whether it is nurse-initiated, physician-initiated, or collaborative in nature.

_____ Administration of Percocet tablets

_____ Recommendations to avoid drinking alcohol before going to sleep

_____ Social work interventions to counsel patient in adjusting to loss of wife

_____ Introduction of guided imagery to aid patient's ability to relax during discomfort

_____ Physical therapy recommendations for establishing routine exercise program

_____ Demonstration of method to change colostomy bag

a. Nurse-initiated

b. Physician-initiated

c. Collaborative

8. Eventually, as Mr. Jungerson's condition stabilizes, he will require education on the skills needed to manage his colostomy. As a nurse you should select interventions carefully. For the nursing diagnosis of *Deficient knowledge regarding colostomy care* related to inexperience, match each of the following descriptions for selecting interventions with the principle on which it is based.

Principle

_____ Expected outcome

_____ Characteristics of nursing diagnosis

_____ Evidence base

_____ Acceptability to patient

_____ Capability of nurse

_____ Feasibility of intervention

Description

a. Select methods of instruction shown through research to be effective in teaching psychomotor skills.

b. Consider the extent to which Mr. Jungerson's pain will affect his receptiveness to teaching.

c. The choice of interventions should be directed toward achievement of self-care.

d. Choice of interventions must be extensive, because Mr. Jungerson is inexperienced and requires thorough instruction on all aspects of care.

e. Confer with Mr. Jungerson on the times when he prefers to be instructed.

f. Review your knowledge of ostomy function and care before beginning instruction.

9. When selecting interventions, you may choose to use the Nursing Interventions Classification (NIC) taxonomy. List three purposes of the NIC project.

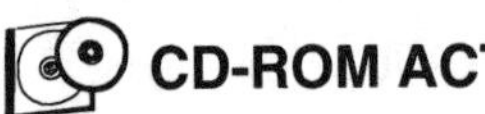

CD-ROM ACTIVITY

Exercise 3—Paul Jungerson, Medical-Surgical Telemetry, Room 602

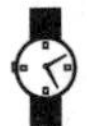

This exercise will take approximately 30 minutes to complete.

In this exercise you will visit Paul Jungerson, a retired postal worker who entered the hospital following a 3-day history of left lower quadrant pain. He had surgery Saturday for repair of a coloanal anastomosis with creation of a diverting transverse colostomy. You may have worked with Mr. Jungerson previously.

- With *Virtual Clinical Excursions—Medical-Surgical* Disk 2 in your CD-ROM drive, click on the **Shortcut to VCE** icon, enter the hospital, and take the elevator to Floor 6.
- Click on the central **Nurses' Station**.
- Find and click on the **Login Computer**.
- Log in to visit Paul Jungerson during the time 13:00–14:29.
- Listen to the Case Overview; then click on **Assignment** and review the Preceptor Note.
- Click on **Nurses' Station**.
- Click on **Patient Care** and select **Data Collection** from the drop-down menu.
- Wash your hands by first clicking in the sink and then on the faucet.
- Enter the room by clicking on the curtain on the right of the screen.
- Review the nurse's assessment of Mr. Jungerson in the following categories: **Initial Observations**, **Vital Signs** (specifically **Pain Assessment**), and **Behavior.**

1. Mr. Jungerson's plan of care includes the following goal and outcome:
   Goal—Patient will achieve pain relief.
   Outcome—Patient will report pain as 2 on a scale of 0 to 10.
   After reviewing Mr. Jungerson's current status, answer the following questions.

   a. What evaluative measures are used by the nurse to determine Mr. Jungerson's pain status?

   b. How would you interpret Mr. Jungerson's status?

   c. What would you suggest in modifying his plan of care?

- Return to the Nurses' Station.
- Find the Medication Administration Record (MAR) on the countertop.
- Click on the **MAR**. Once inside, be sure to click on the tab with Mr. Jungerson's room number—**602**—to access the correct records.
- Review Mr. Jungerson's PRN medication orders.

2. It is now 13:00. Considering Mr. Jungerson's pain status, when can you again administer morphine sulfate?

3. Based on your review of the Assignment data, you recognize that Mr. Jungerson's condition is changing. For each of the findings below, identify how the finding would be evaluated.

Finding	Evaluative Measure
Bowel sounds hypoactive	
Emesis	
Abdomen large	
Temperature 101.2° F	

- Return to the Nurses' Station.
- Click on **Patient Records** and select **Chart** from the drop-down menu.
- Click on **Physician Orders** and read the orders for 13:00.

4. Mr. Jungerson's GI status is changing. Give a rationale for each order listed below. (*Study Tip:* Refer to a pharmacology text if needed.)

Order	Rationale
NPO	
Unasyn 3 g IVPB	
Increase IVF	

5. Based on your evaluation of Mr. Jungerson's clinical status, what might be necessary in regard to his plan of care?

6. Describe two factors you should examine when evaluating an intervention.

LESSON 3

Physical Examination and Vital Signs

Reading Assignment: Health Assessment and Physical Examination (Chapter 32)
Vital Signs (Chapter 31)

Patients: Darlene Martin, Surgery (Floor 4); Medical-Surgical Telemetry (Room 613)
Julia Parker, Room 608

Objectives

- Critique the approaches used in the case studies for conducting a physical examination and measuring vital signs.
- Explain why certain physical examination techniques are used with patients in the case studies.
- Recognize abnormal vital signs and physical assessment findings.
- Discuss how changes resulting from disease or surgical conditions might affect physical examination findings and vital signs.
- Identify assessments required for identifying select nursing diagnoses.
- Identify priority areas of assessment for a specific patient.
- Discuss how nursing therapies might change physical examination findings.

As a nurse, you must acquire and practice the skillful use of a valuable set of tools for assessing a patient's condition: conducting a physical examination and measuring vital signs. Findings from an examination help to determine the patient's needs and the types of nursing therapies most appropriate. After you administer nursing therapies, physical examination and vital sign measurement can help you to evaluate how the patient responds and determine whether the plan of care can continue or should be revised. The exercises in this lesson will give you a clear sense of how physical examination and vital sign measurement become incorporated into a nurse's daily routine and how approaches are individualized based on a patient's history and presenting condition. This lesson also gives you an opportunity to compare examination approaches based on different patients' presenting symptoms.

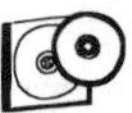 **CD-ROM Activity**

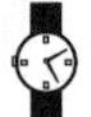 This exercise will take approximately 45 minutes to complete.

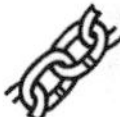 This exercise links to Lesson 14.

Exercise 1—Darlene Martin, Surgery (Floor 4)

- With *Virtual Clinical Excursions – Medical-Surgical* Disk 2 in your CD-ROM drive, click on the **Shortcut to VCE icon**, enter the hospital, and take the elevator to Floor 4. (*Note:* If you need help with these steps, see pp. 5–10 of the **Getting Started** section of this workbook.)
- Click on the central **Nurses' Station**.
- Find and click on the **Login Computer**.
- Sign in to visit Darlene Martin during Preop Care (06:30–07:29).
- Click on the **Nurses' Station** button in the lower right corner of the screen.
- Listen to the Case Overview; then click on **Assignment** and read the Preceptor Note.
- Click on **Nurses' Station** in the bottom right corner of the screen.
- Click on **Patient Records** in the upper left side of the Nurses' Station screen and select **Chart** from the drop-down menu.
- First, read the **History & Physical**.
- Next, click on **Nursing History** and review this section also.

It is important to have a baseline understanding of a patient's condition before conducting physical measurements. This is, of course, not always possible, especially in emergent situations. However, your knowledge of a patient's clinical condition better enables you to interpret the meaning and significance of physical assessment findings and vital sign values.

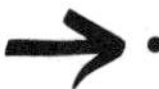

- Click on the **Nurses' Station** icon in the lower right of the screen.
- From the Nurses' Station, click on **Patient Records** and then on **EPR**.
- Enter the password—**nurse2b**—and click on **Access Records**.
- Review all system assessments.

1. The assessment of Ms. Martin reveals a Glascow Coma Scale (GCS) of 15. This would be interpreted as:
   a. disoriented.
   b. unresponsive.
   c. normal.
   d. hyperactive.

2. Once Ms. Martin returns from surgery, the nurse will repeat the GCS. What would be the likely finding immediately postop? Explain.

3. Ms. Martin's peripheral pulses are 2+. How would you categorize that finding, and what is the reason for including this measurement in a preoperative assessment? (*Hint:* Refer to the section on preoperative physical examination in Chapter 49 of your textbook.)

4. On the diagram below, mark with an **X** the locations where you would palpate the following pulses: femoral, popliteal, dorsalis pedis.

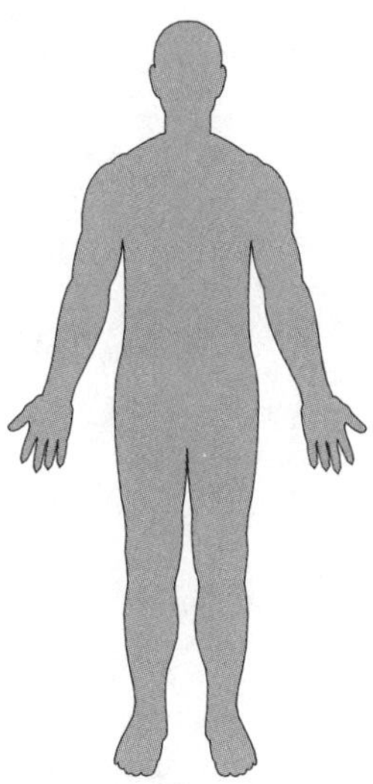

5. Why should you palpate pulses in both extremities at the same time?

6. Which of the following pulses do you never palpate at the same time?
   a. Radial and ulnar in the same arm
   b. Carotid pulse on the left and right
   c. Brachial and radial in the same arm
   d. Femoral pulse on the left and right

→
- When you have finished reviewing all the system assessments in the EPR, click on the **Nurses' Station** in the lower right corner of your screen.
- Click on **Patient Care** from the menu on the left side of the screen and select **Data Collection** to go to Ms. Martin's room.
- Before you enter the room, wash your hands by first clicking in the sink and then on the faucet.
- Enter the room by clicking on the curtain on the right of the screen.
- Click on **Initial Observations** and review the nurse conducting an assessment of Ms. Martin.

7. The nurse tells you in the Initial Observation that Ms. Martin "may seem sleepy." Circle the examination categories below that might most be affected by a patient being "sleepy." Give a rationale for each of your choices.

Abdominal appearance

Lung sounds

Sensory testing

Lymph node palpation

General behavior

→ • Still in Ms. Martin's room, click on the **Head & Neck** area on the revolving 3-D body model. Then click on each assessment option in the menu in the middle of the screen.

• Review all assessments.

8. The abbreviation PERRLA indicates what?

→ • Click on the **Chest & Back** area of the revolving body model. Then click on each assessment option in the menu in the middle of the screen.

• Review all assessments.

9. Observe the nurse's technique for assessing Ms. Martin's lung sounds. On the diagram below, which contains empty circles for the proper auscultation pattern, write in numbers for the actual stethoscope placement used by the nurse.

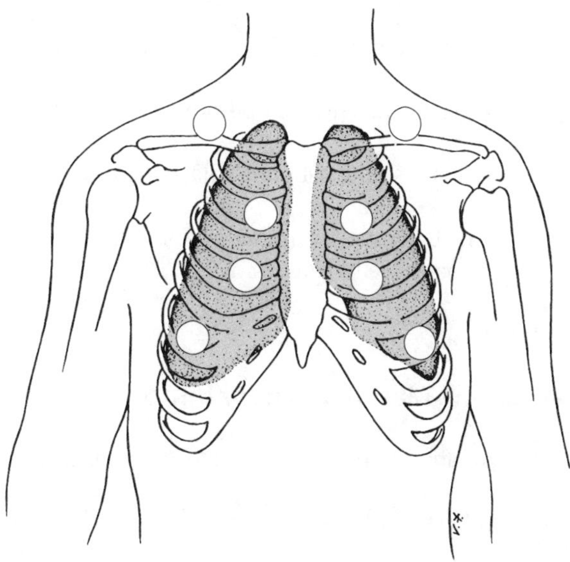

10. The nurse's auscultation of lung sounds was not as methodical as is recommended. However, the nurse did focus attention on the patient's lower lobes. Why is this important in this particular patient?

11. Fill in the blank: When auscultating lung sounds, use the ____________________ of the stethoscope.

12. The nurse documents "no accessory muscle use" for assessment of musculoskeletal status. How is this finding examined?
    a. Palpation
    b. Percussion
    c. Auscultation
    d. Inspection

→ • Click on the **GI & GU** area of the body model. Then click on each option in the menu in the middle of the screen to observe the complete abdominal assessment.
• Review all assessments.

13. Pay particular attention to the photograph of the nurse assessing abdominal appearance. What is incorrect about this photo?

14. Identify whether each of the following statements describing abdominal assessment is true or false.

    a. ________ During abdominal assessment, place the patient's arms across the chest.

    b. ________ When examining the abdomen, assess tender areas first.

    c. ________ Have the patient void before an abdominal examination.

    d. ________ Encourage the patient to place the arms under the head during palpation.

    e. ________ An abdominal examination follows the order of inspection, auscultation, palpation, and percussion.

CD-ROM Activity

Exercise 2—Darlene Martin, Surgery (Floor 4)

This exercise will take approximately 30 minutes to complete.

This exercise links to Lesson 14, Exercise 1.

If you are continuing directly from Exercise 1, sign out from your current period of care and log in again to work with Ms. Martin, this time for the 09:30–10:29 period of care. (*Note*: If you need help, see p. 27 of the **Getting Started** section of this workbook for detailed steps on switching patients or periods of care.) If you are just starting for the day and do not already have the software running, refer to pp. 5–10 of the **Getting Started** section for instructions on entering the hospital, selecting a clinical rotation, and working with patients. When you arrive at Floor 4, sign in to care for Darlene Martin at 09:30–10:29.

- Listen to the Case Overview report.
- Click on **Nurses' Station** in the lower right of the screen.
- Click on **Patient Records** and select **Chart** from the drop-down menu.
- Click on **Operative Records** and review.

1. The anesthesia questionnaire notes that Ms. Martin has an MVP (mitral valve prolaspe). On examination she was found to have a murmur. Fill in the blanks:

   a. If a murmur occurs between S_2 and S_1, it is a __________________ murmur.

   b. Murmurs can be caused by __________________ blood flow through a normal valve.

   c. While auscultating a murmur, the nurse determines its place in the __________________ cycle.

- Return to the Nurses' Station.
- Click on **Patient Care** and select on **Data Collection** to visit Ms. Martin.
- Wash your hands by first clicking in the sink and then on the faucet.
- Enter the room by clicking on the curtain on the right of the screen.
- Click on **Vital Signs**. Then, one at a time, click on each vital sign assessment option in the center menu.
- Observe measurement of all vital signs.

2. The nurse checks the placement of the pulse oximeter sensor on Ms. Martin's finger. An appropriate oximeter site has two characteristics. List each.

3. Which of the following findings in Ms. Martin's assessment can cause an inaccurate pulse oximeter reading?
   a. Low body temperature
   b. Light skin pigment
   c. High carbon dioxide levels
   d. Irregular heart rate

→ • Next, click on the **Head & Neck** area on the revolving figure. Then click on each assessment option in the center menu. Pay close attention to the cranial nerve assessment.

4. The nurse's technique for measuring cranial nerve function was focused on assessing which nerves?
   a. Cranial nerves I and V
   b. Cranial nerves III, IV, and VI
   c. Cranial nerves VI and VII
   d. Cranial nerve II

→ • Click on the **Chest & Back** area of the revolving figure. Then click on each assessment option in the menu in the middle of the screen. After clicking on **Respiratory**, pay close attention the nurse's assessment of Ms. Martin's lung sounds.

5. Ms. Martin is just awakening from anesthesia. The nurse has her turn to her side in order to assess posterior lung sounds. Which of the following normal breath sounds are heard best posteriorly?
   a. Bronchial
   b. Vesicular
   c. Rhonchi
   d. Bronchovesicular

→ • Click on the **GI & GU** area of the revolving figure. Then click on each assessment option in the menu in the middle of the screen.
• Review all assessments.

6. Note the description of the patient's abdominal appearance. This entry is incorrect; explain why.

7. Indicate whether each of the following statements describing abdominal inspection is true or false.

   a. ________ A patient free of abdominal pain will not splint the abdomen.

   b. ________ To inspect the abdomen for abnormal movement, sit to the patient's right side and look across the abdomen.

   c. ________ A round abdomen protrudes in a concave sphere from the horizontal plane.

   d. ________ The presence of a mass on only one side may indicate an underlying mass.

   e. ________ With distention the entire abdomen protrudes and the skin is taut.

8. What is the likely cause for Ms. Martin to have absent bowel sounds in all four quadrants?

9. Fill in the blanks:

   a. To listen to bowel sounds, use the ____________________ of the stethoscope.

   b. It normally takes ____________________ to hear a bowel sound.

   c. Hyperactive sounds are loud, growling sounds called ____________________.

   d. The best time to auscultate bowel sounds is ____________________.

10. Explain why you auscultate bowel sounds before palpation.

CD-ROM Activity

Exercise 3—Julia Parker, Medical-Surgical/Telemetry, Room 608

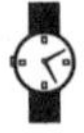

This exercise will take approximately 45 minutes to complete.

If you are continuing directly from Exercise 2 of this lesson, switch patients by logging out and signing in again on the Login Computer (see p. 27 in the **Getting Started** section for help). If you are just starting for the day and do not already have the software running, refer to pp. 5–10 of the **Getting Started** section for instructions on entering the hospital, selecting a clinical rotation, and working with patients.

- With *Virtual Clinical Excursions—Medical-Surgical* Disk 2 in your CD-ROM drive, click on the **Shortcut to VCE** icon, enter the hospital, and take the elevator to the 6th floor.
- Log in to care for Julia Parker during the 07:00–08:29 period of care.
- Listen to the Case Overview.

In the chart provided below, fill in the information you hear from the nurse's summary.

Presenting signs/symptoms:
Patient's perception of health problem:
Surgical treatment:
Pain rating: 06:00 _____ 06:30 _____
Treated with ______________________________ at 06:00
Treated with ______________________________ at 06:30
BP:
Heart rate:
Respirations:
SpO_2
Lung sounds:
Presence of edema: Yes No
Peripheral pulses:

1. Based on the data you gained from the Case Overview, which of the physical examination categories below are priorities for this patient? Circle your answers and give a rationale for each.

Neurologic

Heart

Musculoskeletal

Lungs

Vascular

- Return to the Nurses' Station.
- Click on **Patient Records** and then on **EPR**.
- Enter the password—**nurse2b**—and click on **Access Records**.
- Review the vital signs summary.

2. At 06:00 Ms. Parker's blood pressure was 146/90. What is the patient's pulse pressure?

- Still in the EPR, click on **Cardiovascular** and review the CV findings.

3. The flow sheet indicates that Ms. Parker had cool and diaphoretic skin at 06:30. What might this indicate?

- Return to the Nurses' Station
- Click on **Patient Records** and select **Chart**.
- Review the patient's **History & Physical** (primary and secondary surveys); then review the **Nursing History** (Activity/Rest).

4. Both sections of the record describe findings for assessment of peripheral pulses. Provide interpretations for the following three pulse ratings:

   a. 0

   b. 2+

   c. 4+

5. The record reports that Ms. Parker had no adventitious sounds. Which of the following is an adventitious sound?
   a. Bronchial
   b. Crackle
   c. Bronchovesicular
   d. Vesicular

6. The record reports that Ms. Parker has no neck vein distention at a 45-degree angle. The assessment of the jugular veins is important, especially in a heart patient. Fill in the blanks:

   a. The column of blood inside the internal jugular reflects pressure in the

   ____________________________.

   b. The higher the column of blood, the ____________________ the venous pressure.

   c. Normally, venous pulsations cannot be seen with the patient in the ____________________ position.

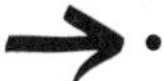

- Return to the Nurses' Station.
- Click on **Patient Care** and select **Data Collection** to visit Ms. Parker.
- Wash your hands by first clicking in the sink and then on the faucet.
- Enter the room by clicking on the curtain on the right of the screen.
- Click on **Vital Signs**. Then, one at a time, click on each vital sign assessment option in the center menu.
- Observe measurement of all vital signs.

7. Observe carefully the nurse's technique for applying the blood pressure cuff. From the list below, circle any steps that the nurse either omitted or performed incorrectly. Provide a rationale for each step you circle.

Palpation of brachial artery

Removal of restrictive clothing

Placement of center of bladder over artery

Positioning arm at heart level

Applying cuff deflated

8. Match each error in blood pressure assessment technique with its corresponding result. (*Note:* You will use one result twice.)

	Error in Technique	Result
_____	Bladder or cuff too wide	a. False low systolic reading
_____	Cuff wrapped too loosely	b. False low reading
_____	Deflating cuff too quickly	c. False high reading
_____	Arm not supported	d. False low systolic and high diastolic reading
_____	Assessment repeated too quickly	

9. Explain why the nurse was palpating Ms. Parker's pulse while counting respirations.

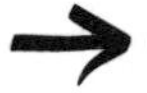

- Next, click on the **Head & Neck** area on the revolving figure. Then click on each assessment option in the menu in the middle of the screen.
- Review all assessments.

10. The summary of findings for the eye examination did not include Ms. Parker's extraocular movements. Write a summary of the nurse's findings as though you were making an entry in her Chart.

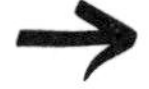

- Click on the **Chest & Back** area of the revolving figure. Then click on each assessment option in the menu in the middle of the screen.
- Pay close attention to the nurse's assessment of Ms. Parker's heart sounds.

11. On the diagram below draw a circle for where you can auscultate heart sounds at the aortic, tricuspid, and mitral areas.

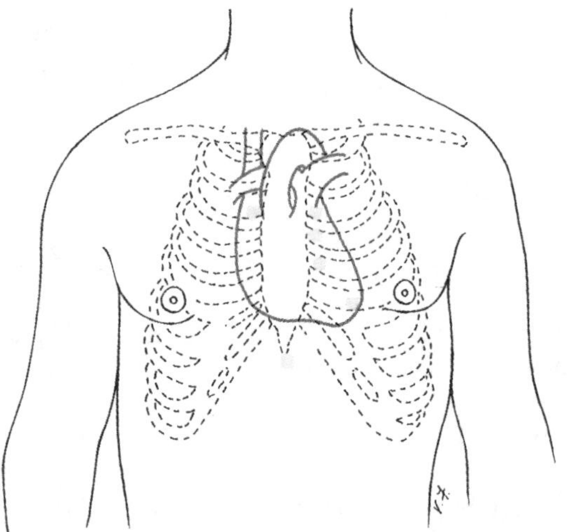

- Next, click on one of the **Upper Extremities** on the revolving figure. Then click on each assessment option in the menu in the middle of the screen.
- Specifically, click on **Vascular** and focus on that assessment.

12. As you observe the nurse palpating pulses on the upper extremity, list the pulses the nurse assesses.

13. Describe the purpose of the Allen's test.

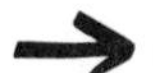

- Click on **Nurses' Station**.
- *Remember:* You must wash your hands before returning to the Nurses' Station. Double-click in the sink and then on the door to the left.
- From the Nurses' Station, click on **Planning Care**; then select **Setting Priorities**.
- Read the Preceptor Note.
- Click on the **Nursing Care Matrix** at the bottom of the screen.
- Review the Nursing Care Matrix, specifically the diagnosis of Decreased cardiac output.

14. Review the characteristics of Decreased cardiac output. Then match each characteristic listed below with its appropriate examination technique(s).

	Examination Technique	Characteristic
_____	Inspection	a. Palpitations
_____	Palpation	b. Arrhythmias
_____	Auscultation	c. Jugular venous distention
_____	Patient's self report	d. Edema
		e. Clammy skin
		f. Dyspnea
		g. Prolonged capillary refill
		h. Decreased peripheral pulses

LESSON 4

Communication With the Patient and Health Care Team

Reading Assignment: Communication (Chapter 23)

Patients: Darlene Martin, Surgery (Floor 4)
Tom Handy, Room 610

Objectives

- Describe levels of communication.
- Identify elements of the communication process while applying a case example.
- Identify examples of nonverbal communication depicted in the case studies.
- Describe aspects of verbal communication.
- Identify therapeutic communication techniques.
- Identify factors that create barriers to communication.

For as long as you are a nurse, experiences with patients will build and mold your ability as a communicator. The ability to communicate well with others helps you to establish the important connection that allows you to deliver quality care to your patients. Excellent nursing is all about relationships. If you are unable to interact professionally and therapeutically, you will fail to understand a patient's needs, concerns, beliefs, hopes, and expectations.

Talking *with* patients, not *at* patients can be difficult. The same is true in regard to patients' families. Communication requires sensitivity, active participation, and an astute interpretation of what people convey through their words and behavior. You must be willing to know a patient and to reveal a bit of yourself in order to establish the trust and confidence necessary to communicate therapeutically.

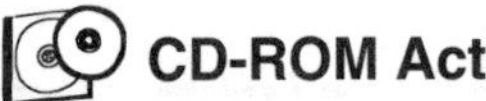

CD-ROM Activity

Exercise 1—Darlene Martin, Surgery (Floor 4)

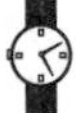

This exercise will take approximately 30 minutes to complete.

In this exercise you will visit Darlene Martin, who has entered the hospital for an elective surgery, a total abdominal hysterectomy. You may have worked with Ms. Martin in a previous lesson.

- With *Virtual Clinical Excursions—Medical-Surgical* Disk 2 in your CD-ROM drive, click on the **Shortcut to VCE** icon, enter the hospital, and take the elevator to Floor 4. (*Note:* If you need help with these steps, see pp. 5–10 of the **Getting Started** section of this workbook.)
- When you arrive at Floor 4, click on the central **Nurses' Station**.
- Find and click on the **Login Computer**.
- Sign in to visit Darlene Martin during the preop interview.
- Listen to the Case Overview; then click on **Assignment** and read the Preceptor Note.
- Click on **Nurses' Station** in the lower right corner of the screen.
- Click on **Patient Care** and choose **Data Collection** from the drop-down menu.
- Wash your hands by first clicking in the sink and then on the faucet.
- Enter Ms. Martin's room by clicking on the curtain on the right of the screen.
- Observe the preop interview.

1. The brief interview is the nurse's initial meeting with Ms. Martin. Describe below how the nurse accomplishes each aspect of the orientation phase.

Sets tone for relationship

Clarifies nurse's role

Expects patient to test nurse's competence

2. The nurse states, "Tell me in your own words why you are admitted." This is an example of:
   a. a focused question.
   b. a closed-ended question.
   c. an open-ended question.
   d. a leading question.

3. As the nurse speaks with Ms. Martin, she is speaking in what zone of personal space?
   a. Personal zone
   b. Public zone
   c. Social zone
   d. Intimate zone

4. List four examples of nonverbal behavior used by the nurse during this initial encounter with Ms. Martin.

   a.

   b.

   c.

   d.

5. In the initial encounter between the nurse and Ms. Martin, the nurse displays nonverbal behavior suggesting she might be a good listener. Using the concepts represented by the acronym SOLER, match each letter with its corresponding behavior.

_____	S	a. Establish and maintain intermittent eye contact.
_____	O	b. Lean toward the patient as you listen.
_____	L	c. Relax and be comfortable with the patient.
_____	E	d. Sit facing the patient.
_____	R	e. Maintain an open posture.

6. Listen to the preoperative interview again. In any interaction there are the basic elements of communication. Identify the element of communication that best fits each of the following descriptions.

   a. ____________________ The nurse needs to gather a nursing history in order to have a preoperative data base.

   b. ____________________ Ms. Martin says, "No, not yet."

   c. ____________________ The nurse asks, "Before we get started do you have any questions for me?"

   d. ____________________ Ms. Martin has concerns about becoming nauseated following surgery.

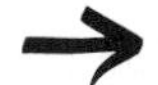

- Return to the Nurses' Station.
- Click on **Patient Records** and choose **Chart** from the drop-down menu.
- Read the Nursing History for Ms. Martin.

7. As you read the nursing history, you will note some quotations from Ms. Martin entered in the record. Using the therapeutic communication techniques specified in the right-hand headings below, provide a response to each of Ms. Martin's statements.

Ms. Martin's Statement	Your Response—Clarifying
"We tend to get along well and work as a team, although we do battle occasionally."	

Ms. Martin's Statement	Your Response—Paraphrase
"I'm just a little nervous about what the pathology report might show, even though we don't expect anything abnormal based on my biopsies."	

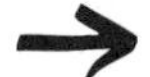

- Return to the Nurses' Station.
- Find and click on the **Login Computer**.
- Click on the **Supervisor's Computer** button and then return to the Nurses' Station. This logs you out of the preop interview period of care.
- Click on the **Login Computer** again and sign in to care for Ms. Martin during the preop care phase at 06:30–07:29.
- Return to the Nurses' Station.
- Click on **Patient Care** and select **Data Collection** from the drop-down menu.
- Wash your hands by first clicking in the sink and then on the faucet.
- Enter Ms. Martin's room by clicking on the curtain on the right of the screen.
- Click on the **Behavior** button on the left of the screen and then on each assessment option in the menu in the middle of the screen.

8. Observe the nurse's assessment of Ms. Martin's behaviors. Specifically, observe the assessment of support. What technique does the nurse use to covey her support towards the patient?

CD-ROM Activity

Exercise 2—Tom Handy, Medical-Surgical Telemetry, Room 610

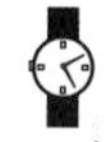
This exercise will take approximately 30 minutes to complete.

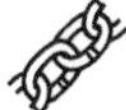
This exercise links to Lesson 5.

Your next patient, Tom Handy, is in the Medical-Surgical/Telemetry Unit on Floor 6. If you are just starting for the day and do not already have the software running, refer to pp. 5–10 of the **Getting Started** section of this workbook for detailed instructions on entering the hospital, selecting a clinical rotation, and working with patients. If you are continuing directly from Exercise 1, sign out from your current period of care and log in again to work with Mr. Handy for the 11:00–12:29 period of care.

Tom Handy is a 62-year-old patient who was admitted to the hospital on Saturday for a right upper lobectomy for lung cancer. You may have worked with Mr. Handy previously.

- With *Virtual Clinical Excursions—Medical-Surgical* Disk 2 in your CD-ROM drive, click on the **Shortcut to VCE** icon, enter the hospital, and take the elevator to Floor 6.
- Click on the central **Nurses' Station**.
- Find and click on the **Login Computer**.
- Sign in to visit Tom Handy for the time period 11:00–12:29.
- Listen to the Case Overview, click on **Assignment**, and read the Preceptor Note.
- Click on **Nurses' Station** in the lower right corner of the screen.
- Click on **Patient Care** and select **Data Collection** from the drop-down menu.
- Wash your hands by first clicking in the sink and then on the faucet.
- Enter Mr. Handy's room by clicking on the curtain on the right of the screen.
- Click on the **Initial Observation** and **Behavior** buttons on the left of the screen and then on each assessment option in the menu in the middle of the screen.
- Observe Mr. Handy during the Initial Observation and during Behavior assessment, specifically noting the nurse's assessment of any signs of distress.

1. As the nurse assesses for signs of distress, Mr. Handy relates important information. Which of the following therapeutic communication techniques would likely result in Mr. Handy discussing more thoroughly what is irritating him?
   a. Offering an opinion as to nature of problem
   b. Using silence
   c. Requesting an explanation
   d. Asking Mr. Handy to clarify what is irritating.

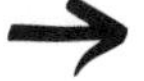

- Continue to observe Mr. Handy's behaviors. Watch as the nurse assesses his understanding.

2. The nurse offers to make herself available to talk with Mr. Handy rather than using a specific therapeutic technique to explore what Mr. Handy is frightened about. At the end of the conversation, the nurse is less therapeutic than she could be. What does the nurse do?

3. List three examples of questions you could direct at Mr. Handy to better understand why he is grumpy and scared.

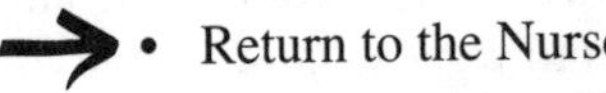

- Return to the Nurses' Station.
- Click on **Patient Records** and choose **Chart** from the drop-down menu.
- Click on **Nursing History** and read, specifically the section on Coping and Stress.

4. Having observed interactions with Mr. Handy and reviewing the history as to the factors increasing his stress, list three outcomes you would plan to achieve in communicating with Mr. Handy.

5. Identify whether each of the following statements is true or false.

a. ________ When communicating with a patient who is cognitively impaired, get the patient's attention prior to speaking.

b. ________ In order to stay focused on the subject matter, do not include family in conversations with the cognitively impaired patient.

c. ________ When a patient does not speak English, use a family member as an interpreter.

d. ________ When assessing a patient with cognitive impairment, ask one question at a time.

e. ________ If a patient is unconscious or not responsive, you may discuss his condition with others in the room.

6. Effective communication with older adults requires a nurse to be aware of any sensory limitations or physical impairments that make communication difficult. For each of the tips listed below for communicating with older adults, provide a rationale based on communication principles.

Get the patient's attention before speaking:

Speak slowly and with good eye contact:

Summarize the most important points of a conversation:

Suppress the desire to finish sentences:

LESSON 5

Patient Education in Practice

Reading Assignment: Client Education (Chapter 24)

Patient: Tom Handy, Room 610

Objectives

- Identify learning principles.
- Distinguish factors that influence a patient's readiness to learn from those that determine the ability to learn.
- Distinguish among the three domains of learning.
- Describe the relationship between learning and psychosocial adaptation to illness.
- Correctly identify components of a learning objective.
- Identify appropriate teaching approaches for the patient in the case study.
- Select appropriate teaching methods based on a patient's learning needs and abilities.
- Describe approaches used to teach patients with special needs or deficits.

As a nurse you will have numerous opportunities to educate patients and their families on ways to manage their health care needs and to promote their level of health. Patient education is one of your most important roles as a nurse. Patients and family members have the right to health education so that they are able to make intelligent, informed decisions about their health and lifestyle. Many patients now receive treatments in their homes and outpatient settings. Effective and appropriate health education is necessary to ensure patients are able to manage their daily health care needs and to minimize the effects of preventable diseases and complications.

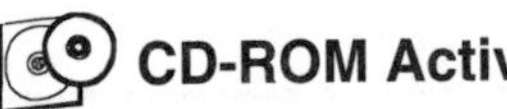

CD-ROM Activity

Exercise 1—Tom Handy, Medical-Surgical Telemetry, Room 610

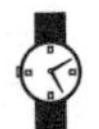

This exercise will take approximately 30 minutes to complete.

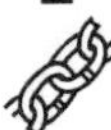

This exercise links to Lesson 4.

In this exercise you will visit Tom Handy, a 62-year-old patient who was admitted to the hospital on Saturday for a right upper lobectomy for lung cancer. You may have worked with Mr. Handy in a previous exercise.

- With *Virtual Clinical Excursions—Medical-Surgical* Disk 2 in your CD-ROM drive, click on the **Shortcut to VCE** icon, enter the hospital, and take the elevator to Floor 6.
- Click on the central **Nurses' Station**.
- Find and click on the **Login Computer**.
- Sign in to visit Tom Handy during the 07:00–08:29 period of care.
- Listen to the Case Overview; then click on **Assignment** and read the Preceptor Note.
- Return to the Nurses' Station.
- Click on **Patient Records** and select **Chart** from the drop-down menu.
- Click on **Nursing History** and review.

1. As you review the Assignment and the Nursing History, complete the following data sheet to assess Mr. Handy's learning needs and his ability to learn.

Expectations of learning:
Learning needs
Information or skills needed:
Motivation to learn:
Behavior
Desire to learn
Learning style preference
Symptoms that can interfere with learning:
Ability to learn:
Sensory deficit
Resources:
Willingness to involve family:

2. This initial source of data (from the Assignment and Nursing History) will be useful to you in planning Mr. Handy's care. What important category of learning assessment is missing in determining how to plan patient education?

- To gather additional information about Mr. Handy, return to the Nurses' Station.
- Click on **Patient Care** and select **Data Collection** to visit Mr. Handy.
- Wash your hands by first clicking in the sink and then on the faucet.
- Enter the room by clicking on the curtain on the right of the screen.
- Click on **Initial Observation** and review the nurse's assessment.
- Click on **Behavior** and then on each of the assessment options in the middle of the screen.

3. After observing the assessments of Mr. Handy's behavior, match each of his behaviors listed below with the learning condition it represents. (*Note:* More than one behavior may apply to a learning condition.)

	Behavior	Learning Condition
_____	Patient is irritable.	a. Patient's knowledge of information to learn
_____	"Doctor said they removed everything."	b. Physical symptoms that affect ability to learn
_____	"I guess I am tired."	c. Family's perceptions of patient's illness
_____	Wishes to speak with wife	
_____	"I still do not understand options for chemotherapy and radiation."	

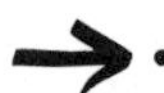

- Return to the Nurses' Station.
- Click on **Patient Records** and choose **Chart** from the drop-down menu.
- Review the Nursing History, particularly the description of the patient's anticipated learning needs.

4. For each anticipated learning need listed, identify the type of learning domain that applies.

Learning Need	Learning Domain
a. Knowledge of purpose and effects of chemotherapy	____________________
b. Skills for managing an oxygen tank or concentrator in the home	____________________
c. Pulmonary rehabilitation exercises	____________________
d. Learning to accept change associated with surgery and threat of cancer	____________________

5. Mr. Handy is having some difficulty dealing with the stress of knowing he has cancer. A patient's psychosocial adaptation to illness influences the ability and willingness to learn. Indicate whether each of the following statements is true or false.

a. ________ When a patient is bargaining in an effort to deal with a loss, the nurse should teach in the future tense.

b. ________ During denial, it is important as a nurse to let the patient know you are available for discussion.

c. ________ The acceptance stage allows a nurse to focus on teaching of future skills.

d. ________ When a patient is angry, the nurse should teach in the present tense and not argue.

e. ________ When a patient begins to experience resolution of grief or a loss, the nurse should continue to introduce only reality.

6. Mr. Handy is a complicated case. He has recently experienced a very sudden loss in health as a result of cancer. At the same time, he has learned the tumor has likely not metastasized. What stage of psychosocial adaptation do you believe Mr. Handy is experiencing? Give your rationale.

7. You have gathered a considerable amount of data on Mr. Handy. It is time to identify nursing diagnoses that may apply to his case. Listed below are defining characteristics for two nursing diagnoses. Match each characteristic with the correct nursing diagnosis.

	Defining Characteristics	Nursing Diagnosis
_____	Patient states, "I still don't understand the options for chemotherapy and radiation."	a. Readiness for enhanced knowledge
_____	Patient is unable to fall asleep.	b. Anxiety
_____	Patient is irritable.	
_____	Patient wants to focus on decisions about proposed treatments.	
_____	Patient has increased wariness or tiredness.	

8. For the nursing diagnosis of Readiness for enhanced knowledge, you must be able to develop learning objectives for the teaching plan. List the four criteria for a learning objective.

   a.

   b.

   c.

   d.

9. Mr. Handy has already expressed interest in learning about chemotherapy and radiation, so decisions can be made about his treatment options. Which of the following learning objectives is written correctly?
   a. Patient will be able to describe risks and benefits of chemotherapy by day of discharge.
   b. Patient will be familiar with benefits of radiation before going home.
   c. Patient will be able to describe benefits of chemotherapy before going home
   d. Patient will be able to describe benefits of radiation by Wednesday, the day of discharge.

10. Considering what you know about Mr. Handy, what teaching approach would you likely use? Give your rationale.

→ • Referring to the Nursing History in the Chart, review Mr. Handy's preferred learning style.

11. Match each of the following instructional methods with its correct description.

	Instructional Method	Description
_____	Group instruction	a. A learner is asked to rehearse a desired behavior.
_____	Preparatory instruction	b. Teacher directly shares information with learner.
_____	Demonstration	c. Teacher instructs number of learners at one time and promotes interaction among learners.
_____	One-on-one discussion	d. Information is provider to learner about a specific planned procedure.
_____	Simulation	e. Teacher poses a problem for patient to solve.
_____	Role playing	f. Effective method for teaching a psychomotor skill.

12. Which of the instructional methods in question 11 do you believe would be suited for Mr. Handy? Give a rationale.

CD-ROM Activity

Exercise 2—Tom Handy, Medical-Surgical Telemetry Unit, Room 610

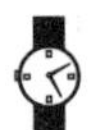

This exercise will take approximately 30 minutes to complete.

In this exercise you will visit Tom Handy, a 62-year-old patient who was admitted to the hospital on Saturday for a right upper lobectomy for lung cancer. You may have worked with Mr. Handy in a previous exercise.

- With *Virtual Clinical Excursions—Medical-Surgical* Disk 2 in your CD-ROM drive, click on the **Shortcut to VCE** icon, enter the hospital, and take the elevator to Floor 6.
- Click on the central **Nurses' Station**.
- Find and click on the **Login Computer**.
- Sign in to visit Tom Handy during the 13:00–14:29 period of care.
- Listen to the Case Overview; then click on **Assignment** and review the updated Preceptor Note.
- Return to the Nurses' Station, click on **Patient Records**, and select **Chart**.
- Click on **Progress Notes** and review.

1. Progress Notes reveal that Mr. Handy is experiencing a change in his clinical condition. When the nurse attempts to instruct the patient, what teaching approach is now appropriate?
   a. Entrusting
   b. Telling
   c. Selling
   d. Participating

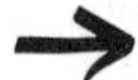

- Return to the Nurses' Station.
- Click on **Patient Care** and select **Data Collection**. (Remember to wash your hands before entering the patient's room.)
- Click on **Initial Observations** and view the interaction between Mr. Handy and the nurse.
- Next, click on **Behavior** and on each of the options in the center menu. Observe each of the assessments.

2. Teaching Mr. Handy will be limited until his confusion and restlessness are resolved. Identify three care activities in which you, as the nurse, could incorporate teaching with nursing care. (*Study Tip:* Review the Physician Orders in the Chart and consider independent measures of care required by Mr. Handy)

3. Fortunately, Mr. Handy is a well-educated man and is able to use the English language readily. However, there are patients with literacy problems who create special challenges for patient education. Indicate whether each of the following statements is true or false.

   a. ________ Functional illiteracy is the inability to read above the fifth-grade level.

   b. ________ Most printed health education material is at a fifth-grade reading level or below.

   c. ________ Patients with illiteracy may be able to understand instructions but not have the ability to problem-solve situations that develop at home.

   d. ________ When teaching a patient who is illiterate, the nurse should provide the most important information at the end of the session.

   e. ________ Reinforce to the patient what is most important to learn at the beginning of the teaching session.

- Return to the Nurses' Station.
- Click on **Patient Records** and select **Chart** from the drop-down menu.
- Click on **Nursing History** and review for information pertaining to sensory deficits.

4. As an older adult, Mr. Handy may require you to adapt your approach to instruction. List three interventions you would use for Mr. Handy.

5. Once you are able to instruct Mr. Handy, it will be important to evaluate whether he successfully learns. Match each of the following evaluation activities with the measurement method it represents.

	Evaluation Activity	Measurement Method
_____	Ask patient to discuss benefits of chemotherapy.	a. Direct observation
		b. Self-report
_____	Have patient correctly attach oxygen equipment and regulate oxygen delivery.	c. Oral questioning
_____	Ask patient to keep record of any side effects from chemotherapy.	

LESSON 6

Documentation Principles

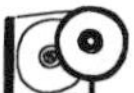 **Reading Assignment:** Documentation (Chapter 25)

Patients: Paul Jungerson, Room 602
Elizabeth Washington, Room 604

Objectives

- Explain the relationship between documented or reported information and the nurse's responsibility for follow-up care.
- Identify elements of quality documentation in written records and verbal reports.
- Write a nursing progress note.
- Identify guidelines used in legal documentation.
- Identify elements to document when communicating a patient's discharge plan.
- Describe principles of home care documentation.
- Explain the type of information to be communicated when a change in a patient's condition occurs.

The reporting and recording of information about patients must be accurate and timely to ensure continuity of health care. The quality of patient care depends on your ability to communicate clearly and effectively with other health care professionals. When aspects of care are not documented or reported, care can become fragmented, repetition of tasks may occur, and therapies may be delayed or omitted. In addition, it is always important to remember that any patient data recorded or reported to other health care professionals must be protected in a confidential manner.

CD-ROM Activity

Exercise 1—Paul Jungerson, Medical-Surgical Telemetry, Room 602

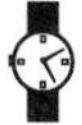 This exercise will take approximately 60 minutes to complete.

- With *Virtual Clinical Excursions—Medical-Surgical* Disk 2 in your CD-ROM drive, click on the **Shortcut to VCE** icon, enter the hospital, and take the elevator to the 6th floor. (*Note:* If you need help with these steps, see pp. 5–10 of the **Getting Started** section of this workbook.)
- Click on the central **Nurses' Station** to enter the floor.
- Find and click on the **Login Computer**.
- Sign in to care for Paul Jungerson at 07:00–08:29.

- Listen to the Case Overview, then click on the **Assignment** button to access the Summary of Report from your preceptor.

1. Use the form below to take notes from the change-of-shift report summarized in the Assignment.

Patient's Name: Admitted:

Diagnosis(es):

Surgery:

Vital Signs: BP ___________ HR _____ SpO_2 _____ RR _____ T _____

Pain Status:

Lungs:

Skin:

Abdomen:

Ostomy:

Dressing: IV:

2. A good change-of-shift report (in this case, the Assignment Summary) should direct you in the care of your patient. Match each of the following elements of Paul Jungerson's Assignment Summary with the corresponding actions you should take.

	Assignment Summary	Actions
_____	Small amount of stool in ostomy bag	a. Check condition of IV site and rate of IV infusion.
_____	Temperature 100.3° F	b. Inspect the color and consistency of stool.
_____	IV in left wrist	c. Check for depth of breathing; determine whether crackles clear with coughing.
_____	Crackles in lung bases bilaterally	d. Inspect IV and wound site for drainage.

- Click on **Nurses' Station**.
- Click on **Patient Care** and select **Data Collection** from the drop-down menu.
- Wash your hands by first clicking in the sink and then on the faucet.
- Enter the room by clicking on the curtain on the right of the screen.
- Click on the various areas of the revolving 3-D body model on the left of the screen and then on each assessment option in the menu in the middle of the screen.
- Specifically, pay attention to the nurse's assessment in the following areas: **IV**, **Respiratory** (within **Chest & Back**), **Abdominal Appearance**, and **Wound Condition**.

3. Based on what you observed, record the nurse's findings for each of the recommended actions below.

Check condition of IV site and rate of infusion:

Inspect the color and consistency of stool:

Check for depth of breathing; determine whether crackles clear with coughing:

Inspect IV and wound site for drainage:

4. Compare the data from the nurse's assessment with the recommended actions.

   a. What information was not collected?

   b. What would you do to correct this problem?

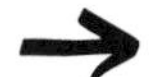

- Return to the Nurses' Station.
- Click on **Patient Records**.
- Click on **Chart**, then **Progress Notes**.
- Read the first Progress Note entered for Mr. Jungerson.

5. Mark on the clock face below the time (in standard time) when Mr. Jungerson's first Progress Note was written in the Chart.

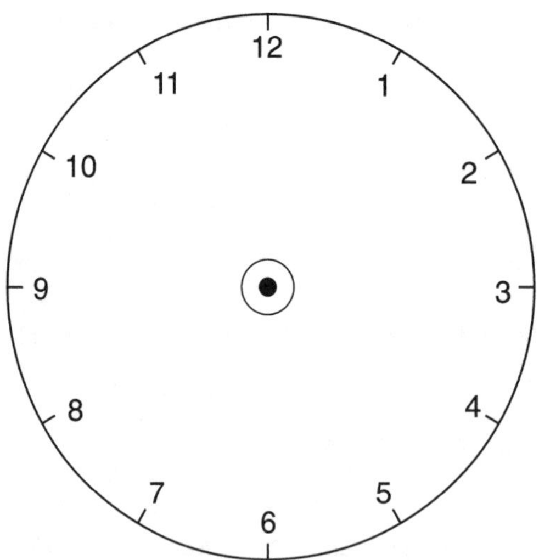

6. Consider the guidelines for quality documentation. Revise each of the following statements from the 06:00 Progress Note in the way you would document them, using the guideline specified after each statement.

"Bowel sounds hypoactive"—Complete:

"Percocet x 2 tabs"—Accurate:

"Tolerable pain relief per IV analgesia"—Factual:

7. Review the Progress Note written for 06:20 by the RN. Convert the SOAP note to a Focus Charting format below.

D—

A—

R—

8. The Nurse's Note written at 06:20 is not well organized. Rewrite the note in a more logical order.

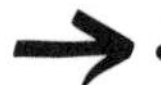

- Click on **Nurses' Station**.
- Click on **Patient Care** and select **Data Collection**. (Remember to wash your hands.}
- Click on **Vital Signs** and choose **Pain Assessment** from the center menu.
- Observe the nurse's assessment of the patient's pain.
- Return to the Nurses' Station.
- Click on **Patient Records**; then select **EPR**.
- Enter the password—**nurse2b**—and click on **Access Records**.
- Go to the flow sheet section for **Vital Signs**.

9. On the flow sheet for Vital Signs, enter the patient's pain rating, and fill in the appropriate cues you observed for Mr. Jungerson.

10. List any additional characteristics of pain the nurse should have assessed for Mr. Jungerson. (*Study Tip:* Review pain assessment in Chapter 42 of your textbook.)

11. Fill in the blanks:

    a. A flow sheet is useful to record routine ____________________ care.

    b. If an occurrence on a flow sheet is unusual, a ____________________

    ____________________ is needed.

    c. A ____________________ is a portable notebook kept at the Nurses' Station for organizing information as a quick reference for nurses.

    d. A discharge summary form is given to the ____________________ at the time of discharge.

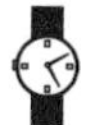

CD-ROM Activity

Exercise 2—Elizabeth Washington, Medical-Surgical Telemetry, Room 604

This exercise will take approximately 30 minutes to complete.

If you are continuing directly from Exercise 1 of this lesson, switch patients by logging out and signing in again on the Login Computer (see p. 27 in the **Getting Started** section for help). If you are just starting for the day and do not already have the software running, refer to pp. 5–10 of the **Getting Started** section for instructions on entering the hospital, selecting a clinical rotation, and working with patients.

- With *Virtual Clinical Excursions—Medical-Surgical* Disk 2 in your CD-ROM drive, click on the **Shortcut to VCE** icon, enter the hospital, and take the elevator to Floor 6.
- Click on the central **Nurses' Station**.
- Find and click on the **Login Computer**.
- Sign in to visit Elizabeth Washington for 07:00–08:29.
- Click on **Assignment** and review the Preceptor Note.
- Click on the **Nurses' Station** button in the bottom right corner of the screen.
- Click on **Patient Care** and select **Data Collection**. (Remember to wash your hands.)
- Click on **Initial Observation** and review this assessment of Ms. Washington.
- Next, click on **Behavior** and then on each of the assessment options in the middle of the screen.
- Return to the Nurses' Station.
- Click on **Patient Records** and select **Chart** from the drop-down menu.
- Click on **Progress Notes** and review the notes for 06:30 on Tuesday and Monday.
- Finally, click on **Social Services** and read the report.

1. Ms. Washington will likely be sent home soon, barring complications. Assume you are going to enter an initial discharge planning note. For each of the standards/criteria for effective discharge planning listed below, record what you know about Ms. Washington.

Family's responsibilities in care

Rehab techniques

Community resources

Signs and symptoms of complications

2. Ms. Washington will likely receive home care until the home health nurse is able to instruct the patient and family on self-care techniques. Explain the primary difference in home care documentation compared with acute care hospitalization.

- Return to the Nurses' Station.
- Find and click on the **Login Computer**.
- Click on the **Supervisor's Computer** button and then click on **Nurses' Station**. This logs you out.
- Click on the **Login Computer** again and sign in to care for Ms. Washington's at 11:00–12:29.
- Click on **Assignment** and review her case summary.

3. Ms. Washington has had an asthma attack. When a patient has a change in condition, a number of criteria must be recorded and reported. For each of the categories below, list three criteria to record for Ms. Washington.

Subjective data

Patient behavior

Objective data

4. What charting system is used to help nurses reduce repetitive recording of normal findings?

5. Following legal guidelines for documentation is the best defense against liability claims. Match each of the following guidelines with its corresponding rationale.

	Guideline	Rationale
_____	Do not erase a chart entry.	a. You are accountable for information documented in chart.
_____	Do not leave a blank space in Nurse's Notes.	b. Maintains secure medical record of your patient.
_____	Chart only for yourself.	c. May appear as if you are trying to hide information.
_____	Do not share your computer documentation password with another caregiver.	d. Another caregiver could add incorrect information to record.

LESSON 7

Safe Medication Administration in Practice

Reading Assignment: Medication Administration (Chapter 34)

Patients: Julia Parker, Room 608
James Story, Room 512

Objectives

- Provide rationales for the selection of medications for patients in the case studies.
- Identify types of medication actions.
- Perform medication dosage calculations
- Describe elements of the six rights of medication administration.
- Explain nursing implications for administering medications.
- Describe potential sources of medication errors.
- Describe the steps to follow in properly preparing injections.
- Identify factors that influence selection of form and route of a medication for administration.
- Explain factors that influence patients' ability to self-administer medications.

Medication administration is one of the more important responsibilities of a professional nurse. Because medications can cause a variety of actions—many of which are nontherapeutic—the safe administration of medications is critical. The busy health care environment poses many barriers to safe medication administration. Thus it is important to learn how to attend to the preparation and administration of medications. You can never be too cautions in administering medications. Always know what medication your patient has been prescribed and why. Know each medication, its purpose, therapeutic action, and common side effects. Be aware of the basic principles used to calculate and prepare medications safely and accurately. Know the effects that medications may have on your patient's behavior and physical condition so that you can properly monitor the patient and evaluate whether the drugs have been effective.

Patient education is an important part of drug therapy. A nurse must make sure that patients know how to self-administer medications safely. This means that patients must know the reason for receiving each medication and how it will affect them physically, cognitively, and behaviorally. Unless patients know the side effects that warn of an inappropriate drug response, they may not consult their health care provider when problems arise. Home environments and daily routines influence how patients take their medications. It is important to problem-solve with patients and families to anticipate possible barriers to safe medication administration in the home and workplace.

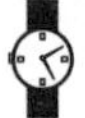

CD-ROM Activity

Exercise 1—Julia Parker, Medical-Surgical Telemetry, Room 608

This exercise will take approximately 45 minutes to complete.

In this exercise you will visit Julia Parker, a 51-year-old patient who was admitted to the Emergency Department with symptoms of a heart attack (myocardial infarction). You may have worked with Ms. Parker previously.

- With *Virtual Clinical Excursions—Medical-Surgical* Disk 2 in your CD-ROM drive, click on the **Shortcut to VCE** icon, enter the hospital, and take the elevator to Floor 6. (*Note:* If you need help with these steps, see pp. 5–10 of the **Getting Started** section of this workbook.)
- Click on the central **Nurses' Station**.
- Find and click on the **Login Computer**.
- Sign in to visit Julia Parker during the 07:00–08:29 period of care.
- Listen to the Case Overview; click on **Assignment** and read the Preceptor Note.
- Click on the **Nurses' Station** button in the bottom right corner of the screen.
- Click on **Patient Records** and choose **Chart** from the drop-down menu.
- Review the **History & Physical**, **Nursing History**, and **Physician Orders**.

1. As you review the Chart information, complete the form below and on the next page. This will summarize key points in Ms. Parker's medical record.

Admitting diagnosis:

Patients' reported signs and symptoms:

Patient's reported allergies:

Patient's weight:

Medications taken at home:

Name	Dose	Route	Ordered Frequency

Preexisting medical conditions:

Additional medications ordered by physician in hospital:

Name	Dose	Route	Ordered Frequency

Nutrition/metabolic factors that may affect medication use:

Patient's preferred method to learn:

Patients method of decision making:

2. After reviewing the medications ordered for Ms. Parker, explain the meaning of the following abbreviations:

SL

SQ

PRN

BID

3. The abbreviation SQ is no longer accepted by the Joint Commission for Accreditation of Healthcare Organizations. What is an acceptable substitute abbreviation?

4. Julia Parker is receiving lisinopril 10 mg PO qAM. What is the rationale for this order? (*Hint:* Refer to your pharmacology textbook).
   a. To control hypertension
   b. To reduce the level of blood cholesterol
   c. To control or relieve pain associated with old fractured ankle
   d. To control the level of blood glucose

5. With a synergistic reaction, the physiologic action of two medications in combination is greater than the effect of the medications when given separately. Review Ms. Parker's ordered medications and list the two drugs designed to act synergistically for her high blood pressure.

6. Explain Ms. Parker's order for MS 2–10 mg IV by answering the following questions.

   a. What does MS stand for?

   b. What is the maximum dose Ms. Parker can receive at any one time?

   c. Once a dose has been given, when is the earliest she can receive the next dose?

   d. What is the advantage of the IV route over the PO route?

   e. What is incorrect in the way this order was written?

7. The order for acetaminophen is 650 mg PO. The medication is available in 325 mg per tablet dose. Use the basic formula below to calculate the amount of medication you would administer to Ms. Parker.

$$\frac{\text{Dose ordered}}{\text{Dose on hand}} \times \text{Amount on hand} = \text{Amount to administer}$$

8. The reason for administering enoxaparin 30 mg Sub-Q q12hr is to:
   a. avoid awakening patient for drug administration.
   b. minimize risk for bruising as a result of injection.
   c. maintain a therapeutic blood level of antithrombin.
   d. administer the drug at the same time docusate sodium is given.

9. Enoxaparin is to be administered subcutaneously. Number the steps listed below in the correct order for a subcutaneous injection.

_____ Check medication order against label on medication.

_____ Perform hand hygiene.

_____ Check patient's name and drug information.

_____ Locate injection site using anatomic landmarks.

_____ Remove needle sheath and hold syringe between thumb and forefinger of dominant hand.

_____ Inject medication slowly.

_____ Pinch skin at site and inject needle at 90-degree angle below tissue fold.

_____ Cleanse injection site with alcohol swab.

_____ Prepare medication from vial/ampule.

10. List two precautions to take when administering a sublingual medication.

11. Match the following descriptions and "rights" of medication administration.

	Descriptions	Six Rights
_____	The nurse determines the patient is experiencing nausea and confers with the prescriber to obtain an order for a rectal suppository instead.	a. Right patient b. Right route
_____	The nurse administers a prn sleeping medication just as the patient is prepared for bed.	c. Right time d. Right dose
_____	The nurse approaches a patient when giving a medication and says, "Please state your first and last name for me."	e. Right medication f. Right documentation
_____	The nurse charts the patient's name, name of medication, and the drug dosage, route, frequency and time given.	
_____	The nurse uses standard measurement devices when preparing a medication.	
_____	The nurse compares the medication container label with the medication record.	

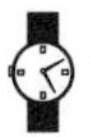

CD-ROM Activity

Exercise 2—Julia Parker, Medical-Surgical Telemetry, Room 608

This exercise will take approximately 30 minutes to complete.

If you are continuing directly from Exercise 1, sign out from your current period of care and log in again to work with Mr. Parker, this time for the 11:00–12:29 period of care. If you are just starting for the day and do not already have the software running, refer to pp. 5–10 of the **Getting Started** section of this workbook for instructions on entering the hospital, selecting a clinical rotation, and working with patients.

In this exercise you will visit Julia Parker, a 51-year-old patient who was admitted to the ED with symptoms of a heart attack (myocardial infarction). You may have worked with Ms. Parker previously if you already completed Exercise 1.

- With *Virtual Clinical Excursions—Medical-Surgical* Disk 2 in your CD-ROM drive, click on the **Shortcut to VCE** icon, enter the hospital, and take the elevator to Floor 6.
- Log in to visit Julia Parker during the 11:00–12:29 period of care.
- Listen to the Case Overview; then click on **Assignment** and review the Preceptor Note.
- Return to the Nurses' Station.
- Click on **Patient Records** and select **EPR** from the drop-down menu
- Enter the password—**nurse2b**— and click on **Access Records**.
- Click on **Vital Signs** and review the summary.
- Click on **Nurses' Station**.
- Click on **Patient Records** and choose **Chart** from the drop-down menu.
- Click on **Progress Notes** and review Ms. Parker's notes for Tuesday.

1. Ms. Parker is continuing to have difficulty with control of her chest pain. If you were the nurse administering nitroglycerine sublingually for her chest pain, what would you include in your preadministration assessment and postadministration evaluation?

2. According to the Progress Notes, the nurse administered morphine sulfate because Ms. Parker received little relief from the nitroglycerine. The morphine sulfate is to be administered intravenously (IV). Match each of the following descriptions with the corresponding IV administration method. (*Note:* A method may match more than one description).

	Description	IV Method
_____	Allows for control of IV fluid intake	a. IV bolus
_____	Preferred when only a small amount of fluid is to be delivered	b. Volume-controlled infusion
		c. Large-volume infusion
_____	Uses piggyback and tandem infusions	
_____	Safest of the three IV administration methods	
_____	Most dangerous method for administering medications	

3. List the three additional "rights" to ensure when administering IV push medications.

4. As a nurse prepares to administer an IV bolus medication, it is important to confirm placement of the IV line. The inability to obtain a blood return suggests:
   a. the IV catheter is too small.
   b. the IV catheter tip is resting against a vein wall.
   c. the patient's heart rate is too slow.
   d. the IV has been inserted into a vein that is too small.

5. The morphine to be administered comes in a glass ampule. Indicate whether each of the following statements is true or false.

   a. ________ Always use a filter needle when drawing up medication from an ampule.

   b. ________ Inject air into the ampule before aspirating fluid.

   c. ________ If air bubbles are aspirated, it is correct to expel the air back into the ampule.

   d. ________ To expel excess fluid in the syringe, hold the syringe vertically with the needle tip up.

   e. ________ Snap the neck of an ampule quickly and firmly toward the hands.

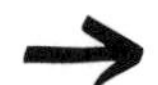

- Return to the Nurses' Station.
- Click on **Patient Care** and choose **Data Collection** from the drop-down menu.
- Wash your hands by first clicking in the sink and then on the faucet.
- Enter the room by clicking on the curtain on the right of the screen.
- Click on **IV**.
- Observe the nurse examining the patient's IV site.

6. Ms. Parker has an intermittent infusion lock in her left forearm. Explain why flush solutions are used with an infusion lock—rather than an existing line—when preparing to give a medication.

7. Which of the following steps are in the correct order for administering a medication by IV push?
   a. Flush IV lock with 1 ml saline; inject medication; flush IV lock with 1 ml saline.
   b. Flush IV lock with 1 ml saline; flush with heparin; inject medication.
   c. Inject medication; flush IV lock with 1 ml saline; flush with heparin.
   d. Flush IV lock with heparin; inject medication; flush IV lock with l ml saline.

8. After administering an IV push medication, the nurse irrigates the lock at the same rate the medication was delivered. Give the rationale for this technique.

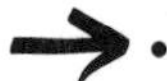

- Return to the Nurses' Station.
- Find and click on the **Medication Administration Record (MAR)** sitting on the counter inside the Nurses' Station. (*Note:* You can also access the MAR by clicking on **Patient Records** and selecting **MAR**.)
- Review the medications administered to Ms. Parker for Tuesday. (*Remember:* After opening the MAR, click on the tab with Ms. Parker's room number—**608**—to access the correct records.)

9. Which of the following medication orders contains an unacceptable abbreviation?
   a. Glyburide 3 mg PO bid
   b. Hydrochlorothiazide 25 mg PO bid
   c. Lisinopril 10 mg PO qd
   d. Zolpidem tartrate 5 mg PO PRN sleep

10. What does a nurse do to determine whether or not a patient requires a PRN medication?

CD-ROM Activity

Exercise 3—James Story, Intensive Care Unit, Room 512

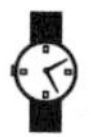

This exercise will take approximately 30 minutes to complete.

In this exercise you will visit James Story, a 42-year-old man who was admitted to the ED with symptoms of end-stage renal disease (ESRD). Mr. Story is currently in the Intensive Care Unit on Floor 5, which can only be accessed from Disk 1. If you are just starting for the day and do not already have the software running, refer to pp. 5–10 of the **Getting Started** section of this workbook for detailed instructions on entering the hospital, selecting a clinical rotation, and working with patients, However, if you are continuing from Exercise 1 of this lesson, you do not have to quit and restart the program. Instead, you may use the bulleted steps below to switch disks and visit Mr. Story. (*Note:* Have Disk 1 nearby before you begin.)

- First, you must log out from your current patient and period of care. To do so, click on the **Login Computer**, click on the **Supervisor's Computer** button, and then select **Nurses' Station**. This logs you out and returns you to the Floor 6 Nurses' Station.
- Now, click and hold your mouse button and move your mouse to the left until you see the open elevator. Click inside the elevator to enter it.
- Once inside the elevator, double-click on the panel of floor buttons to the right of the open door. Then click on button **5** for the Intensive Care Unit.
- The door of your CD-ROM drive should open automatically, and your screen will prompt you to switch disks.
- Remove Disk 2 and insert *Virtual Clinical Excursions—Medical-Surgical* Disk 1 in the CD-ROM drive.
- Close the door to your CD-ROM drive and click again on button **5**.
- When the elevator doors reopen onto Floor 5, click on the central **Nurses' Station**.
- Find and click on the **Login Computer** and sign in for Mr. Story at 07:00–08:29.
- Listen to the Case Overview; click on **Assignment** and read the Preceptor Note, focusing on the brief patient history.
- Click on **Nurses' Station**.
- Click on **Patient Records** and select **Chart** from the drop-down menu.
- Click on **Nursing History** and review.

1. Mr. Story has insulin-dependent type 1 diabetes. This means he has been taking insulin for control of his diabetes for several years. His wife is his caregiver. As the nurse, what would you want to assess in regard to Mr. Story's ability to self-administer insulin?

2. The Nursing History notes that Mr. Story has taken both regular insulin and NPH insulin at home. Which of the following is accurate regarding the action of these medications?
   a. NPH insulin is a rapid-acting insulin.
   b. Regular insulin is colorless or clear in a vial.
   c. Only NPH insulin can be given IV.
   d. Regular insulin is a rapid-acting insulin.

→ • Still in the Chart, click on **Medication Records** and review the orders for Monday.

3. Mr. Story is ordered to receive regular insulin Sub-Q 10 units and NPH insulin Sub-Q 10 units. Number the following steps in the correct order for mixing these two kinds of insulin.

_____ Remove the syringe from the vial of NPH (cloudy) insulin.

_____ Remove the syringe from the regular (clear) insulin after removing air bubbles.

_____ Administer the insulin mixture within 5 minutes of preparation.

_____ Inject air, equal to the dose of NPH insulin, into the vial of NPH (cloudy) insulin.

_____ Return to the vial of NPH (cloudy) insulin and withdraw the correct dose.

_____ Now take the syringe and inject air, equal to the dose of regular insulin, into the clear vial. Then withdraw the correct dose of regular insulin.

4. On the diagram below, mark the sites used for insulin injections.

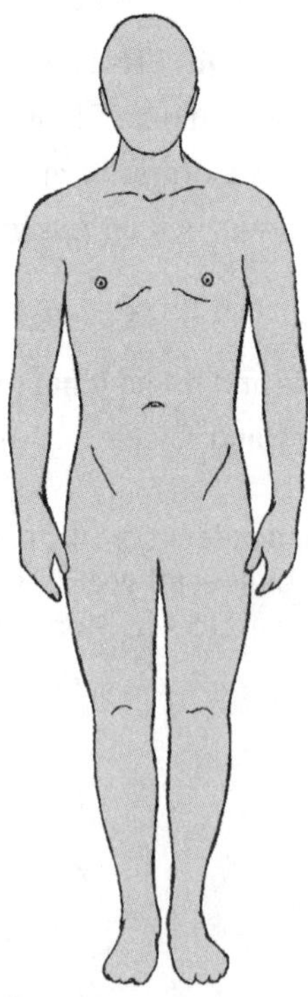

5. Mr. Story is also ordered to receive lanoxin 0.05 mg IV. This medication comes prepared in ampules of 0.025 mg per ml. Compute the correct volume of medication to deliver to Mr. Story, using the formula below.

$$\frac{\text{Dose ordered}}{\text{Dose on hand}} \times \text{Amount on hand} = \text{Amount to administer}$$

LESSON 8

Managing Fluid and Electrolyte Balances

Reading Assignment: Fluids, Electrolytes, and Acid-Base Balances (Chapter 40)
Nutrition (Chapter 43)

Patient: Paul Jungerson, Room 602

Objectives

- Describe the regulation of body fluids.
- Explain the function of electrolytes.
- Describe the processes involved in acid-base balances.
- Conduct an assessment of intake and output.
- Describe criteria for clinical assessment of a patient for fluid and electrolyte balance.
- Describe variables that affect fluid and electrolyte balance.
- Explain factors to include during assessment of the condition of an intravenous site.
- Describe principles applied for insertion of an intravenous catheter.
- Calculate an intravenous flow rate.
- Describe factors to monitor for total parenteral nutrition.
- Identify common complications of total parenteral nutrition.

Fluid and electrolyte and acid-base balances are necessary for the maintenance of health and function of all body systems. As a nurse it is important to understand what physiologic changes occur from fluid and electrolyte and acid-base imbalances, the risks a given patient has for imbalance, and the types of therapies used to reverse imbalance. One of the most important responsibilities for a nurse is to monitor patients closely for fluid and electrolyte or acid-base changes. A patient's condition can change very quickly, thus requiring a nurse's astute observation and timely action.

Competency in the safe and effective administration of intravenous fluid therapy is critical to management of fluid and electrolyte and acid-base alterations. This includes knowing how to correctly establish IV access, monitoring and calculating IV flow rates, and maintaining infusion systems. How well you manage IV infusion therapy may determine your patient's clinical course.

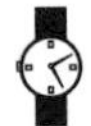

CD-ROM Activity

Exercise 1—Paul Jungerson, Medical-Surgical Telemetry, Room 602

This exercise will take approximately 30 minutes to complete.

In this exercise you will visit Paul Jungerson, a retired postal worker who entered the hospital following a 3-day history of left lower quadrant pain. He had surgery Saturday for repair of a coloanal anastomosis with creation of a diverting transverse colostomy and Hartmann's pouch. You may have worked with Mr. Jungerson previously.

- With *Virtual Clinical Excursions—Medical-Surgical* Disk 2 in your CD-ROM drive, click on the **Shortcut to VCE** icon, enter the hospital, and take the elevator to Floor 6. (*Note:* If you need help with these steps, see pp. 5–10 of the **Getting Started** section of the workbook.)
- Click on the central **Nurses' Station**.
- Find and click on the **Login Computer**.
- Sign in to visit Paul Jungerson for 07:00–08:29.
- Listen to the Case Overview; then click on **Assignment** and review the Preceptor Note.
- Click on **Nurses' Station**.
- Click on **Patient Records** and select **Chart** from the drop-down menu.
- Review the **History & Physical.**

1. Your assessment of Mr. Jungerson should apply critical thinking principles to ensure a complete and accurate database. Your approach to assessment will determine whether an appropriate plan of care can be developed for him. Complete the critical thinking diagram below by writing the letter of each critical thinking factor (on the next page) under its corresponding category.

Knowledge

(1) ____________

(2) ____________

(3) ____________

(4) ____________

Experience	**Assessment Paul Jungerson**	**Standards**
(5) ____________		(6) ____________
		(7) ____________

Attitudes

(8) ____________

(9) ____________

Critical Thinking Factors

a. When you conduct a physical examination of Mr. Jungerson, a focus should be the abdominal portion of the exam.
b. Apply what you have learned in caring for other surgical patients when you assess Mr. Jungerson.
c. Review the surgical procedure for a temporary colostomy.
d. The History & Physical included few details on how Mr. Jungerson has accepted the death of his wife. Clarify this event with the patient and determine how it is affecting his emotional health.
e. Reflect on what you have learned about normal electrolyte regulation and apply this to Mr. Jungerson's clinical condition.
f. Mr. Jungerson is alert and oriented. As you conduct the assessment, allow him to be an active participant in the exam and respect his right to make decisions.
g. Information regarding principles of postoperative nursing care will be useful in assessing Mr. Jungerson's risk for postoperative complications.
h. Use known criteria for normal electrolyte levels and compare these with Mr. Jungerson's actual electrolyte values.
i. Consider theories pertaining to grief and loss when you assess Mr. Jungerson's behaviors and reaction to the loss of his wife.

→ • Still in the Chart, click on **Laboratory Reports** and review Mr. Jungerson's test results.

2. Complete the table below to summarize Mr. Jungerson's key laboratory measurements. Identify and circle any abnormalities. (*Study Tip:* Refer to a lab reference to determine whether Mr. Jungerson has any abnormal laboratory values.)

Lab Value	Saturday	Monday	Tuesday
WBC			
Glucose			
Na			
K			
Cl			
CO_2			

3. Potassium, a major electrolyte and principal cation in intracellular fluid, regulates:
   a. enzyme activities and blood clotting.
   b. water balance and chemical base buffer.
   c. transmission and conduction of nerve impulses.
   d. renal function and sodium balance.

4. If Mr. Jungerson were to continue to have a low sodium level, consider what his clinical picture might look like. List three symptoms of hyponatremia.

5. The movement of sodium out of a cell and potassium being pumped into cells against a concentration gradient is an example of:
   a. diffusion.
   b. osmosis.
   c. filtration.
   d. active transport.

→ • Still in Mr. Jungerson's Chart, click on **Nursing History**. (*Note:* If you are still viewing the Laboratory Reports section, you will need to click on the **Flip-Back** icon until you reach the Nursing History.) Review the history, paying specific attention to the Nutrition/Metabolism section.

6. After reviewing Mr. Jungerson's History & Physical and Nursing History, what do you believe might have contributed to his low sodium level on Saturday coupled with a relatively low blood glucose level?

7. As you conduct a nursing assessment, a number of factors must be considered that can contribute to fluid and electrolyte alterations. Identify whether each of the following statements is true or false.

   a. ________ An older adult is at risk for sodium imbalance because of a decrease in glomerular filtration rate.

   b. ________ A patient's reluctance to cough and deep-breathe postoperatively increases his or her risk for respiratory alkalosis.

   c. ________ Hyperventilation, which can occur with fever, causes a patient to experience respiratory alkalosis.

   d. ________ Patients with cardiac or heart disease have a diminished cardiac output and therefore a risk for sodium retention.

   e. ________ When nutritional intake is inadequate, the body preserves protein stores by breaking down glycogen and fat, resulting in metabolic alkalosis.

8. Fill in the blanks:

   a. Arterial pH is an indirect measurement of ____________________ concentration.

   b. The normal pH of arterial blood ranges from ____________________ to ____________________.

   c. When carbon dioxide increases as a result of metabolism, excretion is controlled by the ____________________.

   d. The two physiologic buffers in the body are the ____________________ and the ____________________.

9. Match each of the following laboratory data with the corresponding acid-base imbalance.

	Laboratory Data	**Acid-Base Imbalance**
_____	pH >7.45 and $PaCO_2$ <35 mm Hg	a. Respiratory acidosis
_____	pH <7.35 and $PaCO_2$ normal or <35 mm Hg	b. Respiratory alkalosis
_____	pH <7.35 and $PaCO_2$ >45 mm Hg	c. Metabolic acidosis
_____	HCO_3 >26 mEq/L	d. Metabolic alkalosis
_____	HCO_3 normal	
_____	pH >7.45 and $PaCO_2$ normal or >45 mm Hg	
_____	HCO_3 <22 mEq/L	
_____	HCO_3 normal or >26 mEq/L	

CD-ROM Activity

Exercise 2—Paul Jungerson, Medical-Surgical Telemetry, Room 602

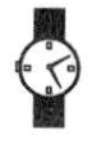

This exercise will take approximately 30 minutes to complete.

If you are continuing directly from Exercise 1, sign out from your current period of care and log in again to work with Mr. Jungerson, this time for the 11:00–12:29 period of care. If you are just starting for the day and do not already have the software running, refer to pp. 5–10 of the **Getting Started** section of this workbook for detailed instructions on entering the hospital, selecting a clinical rotation, and working with patients.

In this exercise you will visit Paul Jungerson, a retired postal worker who entered the hospital for surgery following a 3-day history of left lower quadrant pain. You may have worked with Mr. Jungerson previously in Exercise 1.

- With *Virtual Clinical Excursions—Medical-Surgical* Disk 2 in your CD-ROM drive, click on the **Shortcut to VCE** icon, enter the hospital, and take the elevator to Floor 6.
- Log in to visit Paul Jungerson during the 11:00–12:29 period of care.
- Listen to the Case Overview; then click on **Assignment** and review the Preceptor Note.
- Click on **Nurses' Station**.
- Click on **Patient Records** and select **EPR** from the drop-down menu.
- Enter the password—**nurse2b**—and click on **Access Records**.
- Click on **Intake & Output** to review the patient's I&O summary.

1. Review the I&O record from Tuesday at 02:00 to Tuesday at 08:00. Fill in the I&O data in the table below.

Source of I&O	Tuesday 02:00	Tuesday 05:20	Tuesday 07:15	Tuesday 08:00
Oral fluids				
IV fluids				
IV meds				
Emesis				
Foley				
Liquid stool				
Jackson-Pratt drain				

2. a. Mr. Jungerson's 8-hour total intake from midnight to 08:00 is equal to ______________.

   b. Mr. Jungerson's 8-hour total output from midnight to 08:00 is equal to ______________.

   c. What additional source of output might Mr. Jungerson have that is not listed?

→ • Return to the Nurses' Station.
- Click on **Patient Records** and select **Chart** from the drop-down menu.
- Click on **Physician's Orders** and review all orders since surgery.
- Click on **Progress Notes** and review notes for Monday evening and Tuesday morning.

3. Mr. Jungerson has had an IV of D_5 1/2 NS 20 mEq KCl infusing at 75 ml/hr. This IV solution is an example of:
   a. an isotonic solution.
   b. a hypotonic solution.
   c. a hypertonic solution.
   d. a lipid solution.

4. Explain the likely rationale for potassium being added to Mr. Jungerson's IV fluids.

5. Insertion of an IV requires good critical thinking skills on the part of a nurse. Match each of the following insertion steps with the corresponding scientific principle.

	Insertion Step	Scientific Principle
_____	Check IV solution, using six rights of medication administration.	a. Increases availability of other sites for future IV therapy.
_____	Keep ends of infusion set tubing sterile.	b. Indicates catheter is in vein.
_____	Prime tubing with IV fluid, being certain no air bubbles remain in tubing.	c. Prevents clotting of catheter and keeps catheter patent until it is secured.
_____	Select a vein for IV insertion distal in the nondominant arm.	d. IV solutions are medications.
_____	Prep the IV site with an antiseptic solution and allow the solution to dry.	e. Prevents an embolus entering vascular circulation.
_____	Once catheter is inserted into vein, look for a blood return before advancing catheter.	f. Prevents bacteria from entering infusion equipment and bloodstream.
_____	Once catheter is inserted, begin infusion by adjusting roller clamp for a slow continuous flow of fluid.	g. Allows time for maximal microbicidal activity of agent.

6. Mr. Jungerson's IV of $D_5$1/2 NS is to infuse at the rate of 75 ml/hr. If we assume the infusion set used with the IV delivers 10 drops/ml, the IV should therefore infuse at what rate (drops/min)? Calculate the rate using the formula below.

Drop factor x ml/minute = drops/minute

- Return to the Nurses' Station.
- Click on **Patient Care** and select **Data Collection** from the drop-down menu.
- Wash your hands by first clicking in the sink and then on the faucet.
- Enter the patient's room by clicking on the curtain on the right of the screen.
- Click on the **IV** button on the left side of the screen.
- Observe the nurse's assessment of Mr. Jungerson's IV site.

7. The nurse observes no redness, edema, or tenderness at either the left or right IV site. Match each of the following symptoms with the corresponding IV complication. (*Note:* Each complication has more than one symptom.)

	Symptom	Complication
_____	Redness traveling along path of vein	a. Phlebitis
_____	Pallor around venipuncture site	b. Infiltration
_____	Skin around site cool to touch	
_____	Warmth over vein	
_____	Pain at site	

8. If infiltration develops at an IV site, describe what actions you should take.

CD-ROM Activity

Exercise 3—Paul Jungerson, Medical-Surgical Telemetry, Room 602

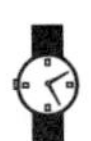

This exercise will take approximately 30 minutes to complete.

If you are continuing directly from Exercise 2, sign out from your current period of care and log in again to work with Mr. Jungerson, this time for the 13:00–14:29 period of care. If you are just starting for the day and do not already have the software running, refer to pp. 5–10 of the **Getting Started** section of this workbook for detailed instructions on entering the hospital, selecting a clinical rotation, and working with patients.

In this exercise you will visit Paul Jungerson, a retired postal worker who entered the hospital for surgery following a 3-day history of left lower quadrant pain. You may have worked with Mr. Jungerson previously in Exercise 2.

- With *Virtual Clinical Excursions—Medical-Surgical* Disk 2 in your CD-ROM drive, click on the **Shortcut to VCE** icon, enter the hospital, and take the elevator to Floor 6.
- Find and click on the **Login Computer**.
- Sign in to visit Paul Jungerson during the 13:00–14:29 period of care.
- Listen to the Case Overview; then click on **Assignment** and review the Preceptor Note.
- Click on **Nurses' Station**.
- Click on **Patient Records** and choose **Chart** from the drop-down menu.
- Click on the Chart tabs for **Physician Orders** and then the **Progress Notes**.
- Review the orders for Mr. Jungerson as they change from Monday 19:10 to Tuesday 13:00. Then review the Tuesday Progress Notes only.

- Click on **Nurses' Station**.
- Click on **Patient Care** and choose **Data Collection** from the drop-down menu.
- Wash your hands by first clicking in the sink and then on the faucet.
- Enter the patient's room by clicking on the curtain on the right of the screen.
- Click on the **GI & GU** area (abdomen) of the revolving 3-D body model. Then click on each assessment option in the menu in the middle of the screen.
- Observe the nurse conduct the complete GI & GU assessment of Mr. Jungerson.

1. Mr. Jungerson is to begin receiving total parenteral nutrition. In this clinical situation, what is the rationale for therapy?

2. The TPN solution will be infusing through Mr. Jungerson's PICC (peripherally inserted central catheter) line, located in his right antecubital fossa. Why is a PICC line needed for the infusion?
   a. PN solutions are highly irritating to small peripheral veins.
   b. PN solutions are viscous and require a large-bore catheter.
   c. PN solutions may cause an allergic reaction, thus requiring establishment of a dependable IV infusion source.
   d. PN solutions are isotonic and infused at a rapid rate.

3. Fill in the blanks:

   a. The measurement of capillary ____________________ testing determines a patient's metabolic tolerance to TPN.

   b. Too rapid an infusion of TPN can lead to ____________________ diuresis.

   c. When a patient is receiving TPN, weight should be measured every

   ____________________.

   d. Sudden discontinuation of TPN can lead to ____________________.

- Click on the various areas of the revolving 3-D model to observe the following assessments: **Head & Neck, Chest & Back, GI & GU,** and **Lower Extremities.**
- Observe the nurse's assessments of Mr. Jungerson.

4. Under each of the assessment categories below, place an X next to any assessment that is relevant to include when assessing for fluid and electrolyte imbalance. In the space to the right, provide a short rationale for each of your choices.

Assessment Categories	Rationale
Head & Neck	
_____ Eyes	
_____ Oral cavity	
_____ Cranial nerves	
Chest & Back	
_____ Respiratory	
_____ Heart	
_____ Musculoskeletal	
GI & GU	
_____ Abdomen appearance	
_____ Bowel sounds	
_____ Urine output	
Lower Extremities	
_____ Integument	

LESSON 9

Nutrition

Reading Assignment: Nutrition (Chapter 43)

Patients: James Story, Room 512
Paul Jungerson, Room 602

Objectives

- Describe factors that place patients at risk for nutritional problems.
- Identify approaches used for nutritional assessment.
- List dietary guidelines for health promotion.
- Identify nursing therapies for improving patients' appetites.
- Describe the selection of appropriate diet therapies for patients with nutritional alterations.
- List steps used in administering parenteral nutrition.
- Identify risks associated with parenteral nutrition.

One of the basic needs that you as a nurse must provide your patients is well-balanced, appropriate nutrition. Without adequate nutrition a patient will not have normal immune function or growth, proper wound healing, or maintenance of metabolic function. Many variables can affect a patient's willingness and ability to eat as a result of illness or injury. Thus, it becomes your responsibility to know how physiologic alterations affect a patient's ability to take in and digest food, factors that alter the patient's appetite, and the effects of therapeutic diet regimens. Anticipating a patient's nutritional needs can be very effective in preventing many complications of disease. The patient, therefore, must be an active partner in helping to select meal plans and approaches that will promote or enhance nutritional intake.

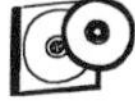

CD-ROM Activity

Exercise 1—James Story, Intensive Care Unit, Room 512

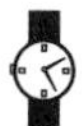

This exercise will take approximately 30 minutes to complete.

In this exercise you will visit James Story, a 42-year-old man who was admitted to the ED with symptoms of end-stage renal disease (ESRD). You may have worked with Mr. Story previously if you completed Lesson 7.

- With *Virtual Clinical Excursions—Medical-Surgical* Disk 1 in your CD-ROM drive, click on the **Shortcut to VCE** icon, enter the hospital, and take the elevator to Floor 5. (*Hint:* See pp. 5–10 of the **Getting Started** section of this workbook for detailed instructions.)
- Click on the central **Nurses' Station**.
- Find and click on the **Login Computer**.
- Sign in to visit James Story during the 07:00–08:29 period of care.
- Listen to the Case Overview; then click on **Assignment** and review the Preceptor Note, focusing on the brief patient history.
- Return to the Nurses' Station.
- Click on **Patient Records** and choose **Chart** from the drop-down menu.
- Click on **Nursing History** and review Mr. Story's history.

1. Based on your analysis of the information in the Nursing History and the Assignment Summary, complete the following dietary history.

Patient name:

Height: Weight:

History of food allergies:

Number of meals per day:

Food preferences:

Special diet:

Appetite:

Taste:

Oral care:

Elimination patterns:

2. Calculate Mr. Story's body mass index. (*Study Tip:* 1 meter is equal to 39.37 inches.)

3. Consider Mr. Story's BMI. Which of the following best describes your findings?
   a. Range recommended for optimal health
   b. Upper boundary for optimal health
   c. Lower boundary for optimal health
   d. High range for risk to acquire hypertension and heart disease

4. Mr. Story has had a poor appetite and is reportedly eating only soup. What factor could contribute to Mr. Story believing he has gained weight?

5. Place an X next to the factors contributing to Mr. Story's anorexia.

_____ a. Nausea

_____ b. Endentulism

_____ c. Insulin

_____ d. Hyperlipidemia

_____ e. Emotional stress

_____ f. Altered taste

_____ g. Shortness of breath

6. List three nursing approaches to use for improving Mr. Story's appetite.

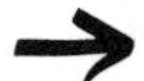

- Still in Mr. Story's Chart, click on **Laboratory Reports**.
- Review the tests and results for Mr. Story.

7. Laboratory tests can be useful in diagnosing nutritional problems. Identify whether each of the following statements is true or false.

    a. ________ A factor that can alter a laboratory test result is a patient's fluid balance.

    b. ________ A common laboratory test used to study nutritional status is hematocrit.

    c. ________ Albumin is a better indicator for chronic disease than is prealbumin.

    d. ________ The condition of diarrhea will increase the body's nitrogen output.

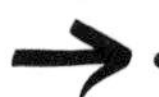

- Now click on the **Flip-Back** icon in the Chart until you reach the Physician Orders section. Review the orders.

8. The physician's order for Monday at 11:00 reads "1800 ADA diet." What does 1800 represent?

CD-ROM Activity

Exercise 2—James Story, Intensive Care Unit, Room 512

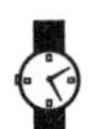

This exercise will take approximately 30 minutes to complete.

In this exercise you will visit James Story, a 42-year-old man who was admitted to the ED with symptoms of end-stage renal disease (ESRD). You may have worked with Mr. Story previously.

- With *Virtual Clinical Excursions—Medical-Surgical* Disk 1 in your CD-ROM drive, click on the **Shortcut to VCE** icon, enter the hospital, and take the elevator to Floor 5.
- Click on the central **Nurses' Station**.
- Find and click on the **Login Computer**.
- Sign in to visit James Story during the 11:00–12:29 period of care.
- Listen to the Case Overview; then click on **Assignment** and review the Preceptor Note.
- Return to the Nurses' Station.
- Click on **Patient Records** and select **Chart**. Inside Mr. Story's Chart, click on **Nursing History**. (Review the entire Nursing History if you did not already complete Exercise 1.)
- Return to the Nurses' Station.
- Click on **Patient Care** and choose **Data Collection** from the drop-down menu.
- Wash your hands by first clicking in the sink and then on the faucet.
- Enter Mr. Story's room by clicking on the curtain on the right of the screen.
- Click on **Initial Observations**, then on **Nutrition**, and then on **Behavior**, observing all assessments, including the additional options that appear in the middle of the screen.

1. It is important for the nurse to develop a nutritional plan of care that incorporates the patient's resources and interest and ability to maintain good nutrition. In addition, the plan should include therapies suited to the patient's needs. Critical thinking applied to planning ensures that a comprehensive and appropriate plan are developed.

   Complete the diagram below by writing the letter of each critical thinking factor under its corresponding category.

Knowledge

(1) ___________

(2) ___________

(3) ___________

Experience

(4) ___________

Planning a Nutritional Plan of Care

Standards

(5) ___________

(6) ___________

(7) ___________

Attitudes

(8) ___________

(9) ___________

Critical Thinking Factors

a. Select diet selections that are consistent with the American Diabetes Association recommendations for dietary exchanges.
b. Apply what you have previously learned in the care of renal patients.
c. Review the dietary sources of fats, fiber, protein, and complex carbohydrates.
d. Plan to have the patient and his wife develop meal plans, taking into consideration Mr. Story's food preferences and financial constraints.
e. Refer to what you know about availability of nutritional resources through home health and community services.
f. Apply teaching and learning principles in your approach to diabetes education.
g. Explore with Mr. Story his feelings about having chronic diseases and whether he might benefit from discussing his concerns with a social worker or clinical psychologist.
h. Select diet therapies consistent with normal nutritional guidelines.
i. Access a listing of all dietary sources to complement Mr. Story's renal and diabetic nutrient requirements.

2. Which of the following diets would likely improve Mr. Story's diarrhea?
   a. Low-residue diet
   b. Low-fiber diet and larger-sized meals
   c. High-fiber diet and smaller-sized meals
   d. Avoidance of acidic foods and sources of caffeine

3. Pictured below is the U.S. Food Guide Pyramid. For each of the food groups, fill in the correct number of servings.

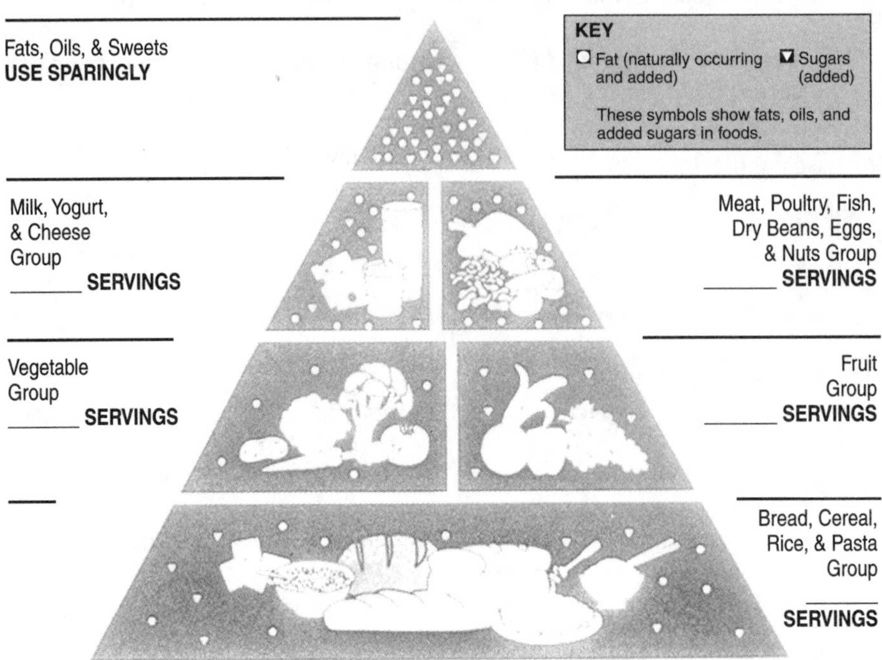

4. Mr. Story was NPO following the procedure to establish a left forearm arterial-venous fistula for dialysis access. His nutrition assessment reveals that he is now taking liquids. Number the following diets in the correct order of progression. (*Hint:* The first answer—clear liquids—has already been chosen for you.

__1__ Clear liquids

_____ Low residue

_____ Mechanical soft

_____ Full liquids

_____ Regular diet

_____ Pureed diet

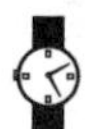

CD-ROM Activity

Exercise 3—Paul Jungerson, Medical-Surgical Telemetry, Room 602

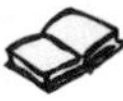

This exercise will take approximately 30 minutes to complete.

In this exercise you will visit Paul Jungerson, a 61-year-old man who underwent a diverting transverse colostomy with Hartmann's pouch on Saturday. You will be observing his clinical case on Tuesday. You may have worked with Mr. Jungerson previously.

If you are continuing directly from Exercise 2, sign out from your current period of care and log in to work with Mr. Jungerson for the 11:00–12:29 period of care. If you are just starting for the day and do not already have the software running, follow the instructions below:

- With *Virtual Clinical Excursions—Medical-Surgical* Disk 2 in your CD-ROM drive, click on the **Shortcut to VCE** icon, enter the hospital, and take the elevator to Floor 6.
- Find and click on the **Login Computer**.
- Sign in to visit Paul Jungerson during the 11:00–12:29 period of care.
- Listen to the Case Overview; then click on **Assignment** and review the Preceptor Note.
- Return to the Nurses' Station.
- Click on **Patient Records** and select **Chart** from the drop-down menu.
- Review the **History & Physical.**
- Next, click on **Progress Notes** and read the notes for Monday at 20:00 and Tuesday at 09:00.

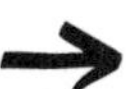

1. The Monday Progress Note written at 20:00 by the physician reports that the patient is nauseated with hypoactive bowel sounds. Which of the problems below might this indicate about Mr. Jungerson's condition? (*Study Tip:* In Chapter 49 of your textbook, read about postoperative complications.)
   a. Wound infection
   b. Atelectasis
   c. Paralytic ileus
   d. Hemorrhage

→
- Return to the Nurses' Station.
- Click on **Patient Care** and select **Data Collection** from the drop-down menu. (Remember to wash your hands.)
- Click on and review the **Initial Observation** and **Nutrition** assessments.
- Click on the **GI & GU** area of the 3-D model and review Mr. Jungerson's status.
- Return to the Nurses' Station.
- Click on **Patient Records** and choose **Chart** from the drop-down menu.
- Click on **Physician Orders** and review the orders for Monday at 19:10 and Tuesday at 09:00.

2. Mr. Jungerson is to receive total parenteral nutrition (TPN). Identify whether each of the following statements is true or false.

 a. ________ Parenteral solutions with high osmolality must be infused into a large-diameter central vein.

 b. ________ The goal of TPN therapy is to move toward use of the GI tract.

 c. ________ An initial infusion rate of TPN is usually 90 ml/hr.

 d. ________ The concentrated glucose in TPN can cause a change in magnesium and phosphorus levels.

 e. ________ A normal lipid emulsion has an oily layer on the surface.

 f. ________ If a TPN infusion falls behind, increase the flow rate to ensure correct 24-hour total infusion.

3. Total parenteral nutrition can result in a number of complications. Match each of the following complications with its proper method for assessment.

	Method for Assessment	Complication
_____	Observe patient's respirations and confer with MD about chest x-ray findings.	a. Catheter sepsis b. Hyperglycemia
_____	Measure patient's temperature and send blood specimen for culture test.	c. Pneumothorax d. Thrombosis of central vein
_____	Ask whether patient senses excess thirst or headache and note frequency of urination.	
_____	Palpate neck and arm for edema; ask whether area of swelling is painful.	

4. Explain the rationale for increasing the rate of TPN infusion gradually.

5. To prevent infection, the nurse should change the infusion tubing of a TPN line with lipids every 24 hours. Why?
 a. Lipids can change the patient's immune function.
 b. A TPN catheter is usually a small-bore catheter that easily becomes occluded.
 c. The high concentration of glucose and lipids promotes growth of microorganisms.
 d. Changes in mineral levels alter the immune response.

LESSON 10

Comfort

Reading Assignment: Comfort (Chapter 42)

Patients: Julia Parker, Room 608
Darlene Martin, Surgery and PACU (Floor 4); Medical-Surgical Telemetry, Room 613
James Story, Room 512

Objectives

- Based on presenting symptoms, describe the types of pain experienced by patients in the case studies.
- Describe the physiologic responses to expect when a patient has pain.
- Conduct a pain assessment.
- Identify the rationale for the physical assessment measures a nurse selects when a person has pain.
- Identify nonverbal responses to pain.
- Apply critical thinking to the assessment of patients in pain.
- Select nursing interventions appropriate for patients in the case studies.
- Evaluate the effects of interventions for pain relief.

Pain is the most common reason people seek health care. Your ability as a nurse to provide comfort for patients requires being willing to accept and understand their pain experience. Pain is one of the least understood of symptoms, because it is unique for each patient. Basic to successful nursing practice is the ability to select appropriate measures to help relieve pain and to enable patients to live more productive and satisfying lives.

The nurse, patient, family, and primary care provider must collaborate to find the most effective approaches to pain control. Both pharmacologic and nonpharmacologic pain therapies can prove to be very effective when used alone or together in the correct situation. You will learn to partner closely with patients in selecting pain therapies and in then determining their efficacy. Effective pain management reduces physical discomforts but also improves quality of life.

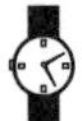

CD-ROM Activity

Exercise 1—Julia Parker, Medical-Surgical Telemetry, Room 608

This exercise will take approximately 45 minutes to complete.

In this exercise you will visit Julia Parker, a 51-year-old patient who was admitted to the emergency department with symptoms of a heart attack (myocardial infarction). You may have worked with Ms. Parker previously if you already completed Lesson 7.

- With *Virtual Clinical Excursions—Medical-Surgical* Disk 2 in your CD-ROM drive, click on the **Shortcut to VCE** icon, enter the hospital, and take the elevator to Floor 6. (*Note:* If you need help with these steps, see pp. 5–10 of the **Getting Started** section of this workbook.)
- Click on the central **Nurses' Station**.
- Find and click on the **Login Computer**.
- Sign in to visit Julia Parker during the 07:00–08:29 period of care.
- Listen to the Case Overview; then click on **Assignment** and read the Preceptor Note.
- Return to the Nurses' Station by clicking on the button in the bottom right corner of the screen.
- Click on **Patient Care** and select **Data Collection** from the drop-down menu.
- Wash your hands by first clicking in the sink and then on the faucet.
- Enter the room by clicking on the curtain on the right of the screen.
- Click on **Initial Observations** and observe the nurse and patient during this assessment.
- Next, click on **Vital Signs** and select **Pain Assessment** from the center menu.

1. Complete the pain assessment chart below.

Onset:	
Duration:	
Location:	
Patient's perception of cause of pain:	
Intensity—06:00:	06:30:
Quality:	
Relief measures:	

2. Based on your observation of Ms. Parker's pain assessment, her pain can best be described as:
   a. radiating.
   b. referred.
   c. superficial.
   d. neuropathic.

3. How might a clearer sense of the location of Ms. Parker's pain been determined by the nurse?

4. Ms. Parker's pain is acute pain from myocardial infarction, resulting from obstruction of blood flow to the heart muscle. In the list below, place an X next to each characteristic that applies to acute pain.

_____ a. Lasts longer than anticipated

_____ b. Short duration

_____ c. Caused by injury healed long ago

_____ d. Resolves with or without treatment

_____ e. Protective in nature

_____ f. Frequently associated with hopelessness

_____ g. Has identifiable cause

→ • Return to the Nurses' Station.
- Click on the **Login Computer**.
- Select the **Supervisor's Computer** and then return to Nurses' Station. This logs you out of the current period of care.
- Click on the **Login Computer** and log in once more to work with Ms. Parker.
- This time, select the 11:00–12:29 period of care.
- Return to the Nurses' Station.
- Click on **Patient Care** and select **Data Collection** from the drop-down menu. (Don't forget to wash your hands.)
- Click on the **Vital Signs** button and then on **Pain Assessment** to observe the assessment of Ms. Parker's pain.
- Next, click on **Behavior** and on each subcategory in the center menu.

5. As you observed Ms. Parker's behaviors, you should have noted several nonverbal expressions of pain. List three behaviors you observed.

6. Suppose that the nurse, after assessing Ms. Parker's pain, decided to implement relaxation exercises. What would be your response?

7. Based on the nature of Ms. Parker's pain, which of the following nonpharmacologic measures for pain relief might be effective?
   a. Repositioning patient anatomically
   b. Administering herbal remedies
   c. Initiating guided imagery
   d. Applying cold compresses

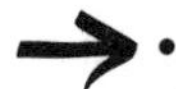

- Return to the Nurses' Station.
- Find the MAR on the desk.
- Click on the **MAR** and review Ms. Parker's PRN medication orders. (*Remember:* To access the correct records, you must click on the tab with Ms. Parker's room number—**608**.)

8. At 6:30, when Ms. Parker reported pain at a level of 8 out of 10, which analgesic was most appropriate to administer? Why?

9. Morphine sulfate is an opioid analgesic. What should the nurse monitor for after administering this drug to Ms. Parker?
   a. Blood pressure
   b. Respiratory rate
   c. Sedation
   d. Urine output

10. Frequently, a primary care provider will order more than one analgesic. Indicate whether each of the following principles for administering analgesics is true or false.

    a. ________ A nonopioid cannot be given with an opioid.

    b. ________ Avoid giving intramuscular analgesics to older adults.

    c. ________ Sustained-release oral analgesics are useful when given PRN for chronic pain.

    d. ________ Avoid combinations of opioids in older adults.

CD-ROM Activity

Exercise 2—Darlene Martin, Surgery (Floor 4)

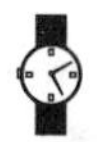

This exercise will take approximately 45 minutes to complete.

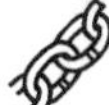

This exercise links to Lesson 14.

In this exercise you will care for Darlene Martin, a 49-year-old female who is to undergo an elective hysterectomy because of a history of fibroids. You may have worked with Ms. Martin in a previous lesson.

- With *Virtual Clinical Excursions—Medical-Surgical* Disk 2 in your CD-ROM drive, click on the **Shortcut to VCE** icon, enter the hospital, and take the elevator to Floor 4.
- Click on the central **Nurses' Station**.
- Find and click on the **Login Computer**.
- Sign in to visit Darlene Martin during Preop Interview.
- Listen to the Case Overview; then click on **Assignment** and read the Preceptor Note.
- Next, go to the Nurses' Station.
- Click on **Patient Care** and select **Data Collection**.
- Wash your hands by first clicking in the sink and then on the faucet.
- Enter the room by clicking on the curtain on the right of the screen.
- Click on **Initial Observations** and observe the nurse and patient during this interaction.

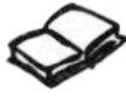

1. In preparation for Ms. Martin's surgery, what should the nurse know so that she can properly inform the patient about any anticipated pain? (*Study Tip:* Read Chapter 49 in your textbook.)

2. Patient-controlled analgesia (PCA) is one analgesic delivery method frequently used postoperatively. The best time to educate a patient about PCA is:
   a. on the surgical unit just before the patient administers the first dose.
   b. when the patient reaches the recovery room.
   c. during the preoperative visit to the surgical center.
   d. in the PACU just before entering the operating room.

3. Indicate whether each of the following statements is true or false.

   a. ________ The goal of PCA is to maintain a constant blood plasma level of analgesic.

   b. ________ A PCA system delivers no more than a specified number of doses either every hour or every 4 hours.

   c. ________ A loading dose is the prescribed amount of analgesic added to the IV pump prior to administration.

   d. ________ Family members can be helpful by pushing the PCA dose delivery button for a patient.

   e. ________ In an opioid-naïve patient increase the demand or basal dose.

→ • Return to the Nurses' Station.
- Click **Patient Records** and select **Chart** from the drop-down menu.
- Click on **Nursing History** and review.

4. Ms. Martin has a history of knee pain. List two precautions the nurse should explain to her about using ice as a therapy.

5. Knowing that activity aggravates Ms. Martin's knee pain, how might this information be useful in planning the patient's pain management postoperatively?

→ • Return to the Nurses' Station.
- Click on the **Login Computer** and then on the **Supervisor's Computer** button. This logs you out of the current period of care.
- Find and click inside the open elevator.
- Go to Floor 6 to visit Ms. Martin postoperatively.
- Click on the central **Nurses' Station**.
- Find and click on the **Login Computer**.
- Sign in to visit Darlene Martin during the 11:00–12:29 period of care.
- Listen to the Case Overview.

6. After listening to the Case Overview, list three possible sources of discomfort that Ms. Martin is likely to experience postoperatively.

7. Removal of painful stimuli is an effective nonpharmacologic method for pain relief. Based on the sources of discomfort Ms. Martin is likely to experience, list three appropriate nursing interventions to remove painful stimuli.

8. Relaxation is another effective pain-relief strategy that can reduce surgical incision discomfort. Match each of the following descriptions of relaxation techniques with the guiding principle.

	Principle	Description
_____	Creates sensation of removing all discomfort	a. Explain the sensations patient will experience during relaxation.
_____	Combined with contraction and relaxation of muscles, this maximizes relaxation	b. Have the patient sit with legs separated and arms at the sides.
_____	Enables patient to use as feedback	c. Have patient attend to areas of tension in the body.
_____	Helps patient to focus on replacing tense area with warmth	d. Have patient locate muscular tension, think about how it feels, tense muscles fully, and then relax.
_____	Puts patient in the natural anatomic position for relaxation	e. Have patient establish controlled diaphragmatic breathing.

- Go to the Nurses' Station.
- Click on **Patient Care** and choose **Data Collection** from the drop-down menu.
- Wash your hands by first clicking in the sink and then on the faucet.
- Enter the room by clicking on the curtain on the right of the screen.
- Click on **Initial Observations** and observe the nurse and patient during this interaction.
- Next, click on **Vital Signs** and then on **Pain Assessment**. Observe.
- Now click on **Behavior** and select **Activity** from the list of subcategories in the center menu. Again, observe the assessment.

9. The nurse tells Ms. Martin that the plan is to have her up on the side of the bed by the afternoon. The best time to administer an analgesic to Ms. Martin would be:
   a. now, so that she has less time to anticipate and worry about the procedure.
   b. before attempting to get her up, so that the peak effect of the analgesic occurs when she is sitting.
   c. just before getting her up to the side of the bed.
   d. once she is positioned on the side of the bed.

10. When you observe the nurse helping Ms. Martin to turn during the Activity assessment, what nonverbal expression of discomfort does the patient show?
    a. Splinting
    b. Groaning
    c. Bent posture
    d. Crying

11. In the Case Overview you learned that Ms. Martin is to have an IVP and CBC in the morning. What interventions would be appropriate to help the patient with these possible painful procedures?

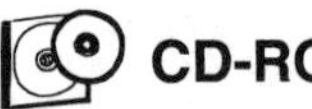

CD-ROM Activity

Exercise 3—James Story, Intensive Care Unit, Room 512

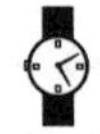

This exercise will take approximately 30 minutes to complete.

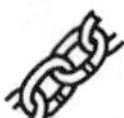

This exercise links to Lesson 9.

In this exercise you will visit James Story, a 42-year-old man who was admitted to the emergency department with symptoms of end-stage renal disease (ESRD). You may have worked with Mr. Story previously.

- With *Virtual Clinical Excursions—Medical-Surgical* Disk 1 in your CD-ROM drive, click on the **Shortcut to VCE** icon, enter the hospital, and take the elevator to Floor 5. (*Note:* If you need help with these steps, see pp. 5–10 of the **Getting Started** section of this workbook.
- Click on the central **Nurses' Station**.
- Find and click on the **Login Computer**.
- Sign in to visit James Story during the 09:00–10:29 period of care.
- Listen to the Case Overview; then click on **Assignment** and read the Preceptor Note.
- Return to the Nurses' Station by clicking on the button in the bottom right corner of the screen.
- Click on **Patient Records** and select **Chart** from the drop-down menu.
- Click on **Nursing History** and review this section.

1. Based on your review of Mr. Story's Nursing History, place an X next to each of the following factors that will affect his pain perception.

    _____ a. Neuropathy

    _____ b. Anxiety

    _____ c. Body build

    _____ d. Social support

    _____ e. Age

- Return to the Nurses' Station.
- Click on **Patient Care** and choose **Data Collection** from the drop-down menu.
- Wash your hands by first clicking in the sink and then on the faucet.
- Enter the room by clicking on the curtain on the right of the screen.
- Inside the room, click on the appropriate buttons to observe the nurse's assessment of Mr. Story in the following categories and subcategories: **Initial Observations, Vital Signs (Pain Assessment), Upper Extremities (Integumentary)**, and **Behavior (Signs of Distress).**

2. The nurse uses a rating scale to have Mr. Story describe the intensity of his pain. Identify two situations when a numerical pain scale works best.

3. When using a pain scale, you should:
   a. always use the same scale for the same patient.
   b. use a scale to compare the pain of one patient with that of another.
   c. have the patient draw a scale on paper.
   d. only assess the current pain level experienced by the patient.

4. Based on your observation of Mr. Story, the pain in his arms can best be described as:
   a. visceral.
   b. idiopathic.
   c. chronic.
   d. somatic.

5. What position might help to alleviate some of Mr. Story's discomfort?

6. List the nonverbal expressions of pain you noticed Mr. Story use during your observation of the nurse's assessment.

7. Mr. Story is experiencing acute discomfort and has a number of chronic conditions affecting his sense of well-being. Critical thinking applied to assessment enables a nurse to develop a relevant and comprehensive plan of care. Complete the following critical thinking diagram for assessment of Mr. Story's situation.

Knowledge

(1) ____________

(2) ____________

(3) ____________

Experience

(4) ____________

(5) ____________

Assessment
James Story

Standards

(6) ____________

(7) ____________

Attitudes

(8) ____________

Critical Thinking Factors

a. Consider the extent that Mr. Story's coping style influences his ability to deal with pain.
b. When administering a pain scale, be sure the patient can see the scale and understand how it is to be used.
c. Previous time spent in caring for patients with acute pain will assist you in recognizing Mr. Story's nonverbal behaviors.
d. Apply pain management guidelines from the American Pain Society.
e. Review the pathology of neuropathic pain.
f. Accept the patient's report of pain and do not make judgments as to whether the intensity is actually less than reported.
g. If you have ever had an injury or ailment causing pain, consider how you expressed your discomfort.
h. Review the pharmacologic actions of analgesics.

LESSON 11

Oxygenation

Reading Assignment: Oxygenation (Chapter 39)

Patients: Elizabeth Washington, Room 604
Tom Handy, Room 610

Objectives

- Identify the relationship of cardiac and respiratory alterations.
- Identify the influence physiologic changes in oxygenation have on a patient's clinical condition.
- Describe factors that normally influence oxygenation.
- Assess the oxygenation status of patients in the case studies.
- Identify nursing diagnoses that apply to patients in the case studies.
- Develop a nursing plan of care for a case study patient.
- Explain the rationale for use of specific nursing interventions for patients in the case studies.
- Evaluate the condition of a patient with an oxygenation alteration.

CD-ROM Activity

Exercise 1—Elizabeth Washington, Medical-Surgical Telemetry, Room 604

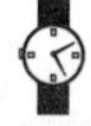
This exercise will take approximately 45 minutes to complete.

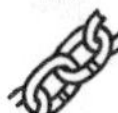
This exercise links to Lesson 13.

Elizabeth Washington was admitted to the ED following an automobile accident. She suffered a broken hip from the accident and has undergone an open reduction and internal fixation of the hip. She also has a history of asthma. You may have worked with Ms. Washington in a previous lesson.

- With *Virtual Clinical Excursions—Medical-Surgical* Disk 2 in your CD-ROM drive, click on the **Shortcut to VCE** icon, enter the hospital, and take the elevator to Floor 6.
- Click on the central **Nurses' Station**.
- Find and click on the **Login Computer**.
- Sign in to visit Elizabeth Washington during the 07:00–08:29 period of care.
- Listen to the Case Overview; then click on **Assignment** and read the Preceptor Note.

- Return to the Nurses' Station by clicking on the button in the bottom right corner of the screen.
- Click on **Patient Records** and select **Chart** from the drop-down menu.
- Review the patient's **History & Physical.**

1. The care of a patient with potential oxygenation alterations requires a thorough health assessment. For each of the findings from Ms. Washington's examination listed below, identify the assessment technique used.

Findings	Assessment Technique
No stridor	
Mucosa pink in color	
Chest wall expansion symmetrical	
Breath sounds clear	
No substernal retractions	

2. Ms. Washington's SpO_2 was normal at 95%. An abnormal SpO_2 indicates:
   a. abnormal alveolar ventilation.
   b. an increase in hemoglobin levels.
   c. central cyanosis.
   d. decreased cardiac output.

3. Match each of the following conditions with its definition.

	Definition	Condition
_____	Collapse of alveoli that prevents normal respiratory exchange of O_2 and CO_2	a. Myocardial ischemia
_____	Deviation from normal sinus heart rhythm	b. Hyperventilation
_____	Insufficient supply of blood to the myocardium from the coronary arteries	c. Atelectasis
_____	Level of ventilation in excess of that required to eliminate normal venous CO_2	d. Hypoxia
_____	Inadequate tissue oxygenation at the cellular level	e. Dysrhythmia

4. According to the History & Physical, Ms. Washington was on several different medications at home. The three medications listed below are aimed at treating her asthma. Match each medication with its classification and physiologic effect on respirations. (*Study Tip:* Refer to your pharmacology text.)

	Medication	**Classification/Effect**
_____	Montelukast Na	a. Bronchodilator; reduces airway resistance
_____	Cetirizine	b. Leuokotriene antagonist; reduces mucus secretion and inflammation
_____	Albuterol	c. Antihistamine; provides palliative relief through drying of secretions

→ • While still in the Chart, click on and review Ms. Washington's **Laboratory Reports**.

5. From Sunday to Monday there were changes in Ms. Washington's hematocrit and hemoglobin levels. What is Ms. Washington at risk for as a result of these changes? What is the reason for the drop in these two values?

→ • Still in the Chart, click on the **Flip-Back** icon until you reach Ms. Washington's **Nursing History**. Review.

6. When you know a patient has a chronic health problem such as asthma, your assessment should include consideration of all factors that may potentially affect oxygenation. This allows you to consider the patient's preventive and/or health promotion needs. For each risk factor listed below, place an X in the Yes or No column to identify Ms. Washington's risks for oxygenation alterations.

Risk Factor	**Yes**	**No**
a. Has a history of smoking		
b. Nutritionally at risk for anemia		
c. Follows exercise plan that improves oxygen consumption		
d. Drinks excessive amount of alcohol		

7. Because of Ms. Washington's history of asthma, it is important to minimize her risk for infection. Identify two approaches you might recommend for her to avoid respiratory infection.

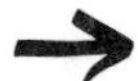

- Return to the Nurses' Station.
- Click on **Patient Care** and choose **Data Collection** from the drop-down menu.
- Wash your hands by first clicking in the sink and then on the faucet.
- Enter the room by clicking on the curtain on the right of the screen.
- Click on the various buttons and parts of the 3-D body model to observe the complete physical examination of Ms. Washington. Pay particular attention to the **Initial Observations** and **Chest & Back** assessments.

8. During the Initial Observations, what position does Ms. Washington assume? How does this position affect her pulmonary function?

9. Ms. Washington reportedly has used an incentive spirometer during her postoperative recovery. Fill in the blanks in the following statements.

   a. Incentive spirometry promotes _______________ ___________________ by providing visual feedback.

   b. Postoperatively, _______________ is a factor that commonly reduces a patient's inspiratory capacity.

   c. When using a flow-oriented incentive spirometer, instruct the patient to inhale

   ____________________ and ____________________.

CD-ROM Activity

Exercise 2—Elizabeth Washington, Medical-Surgical Telemetry, Room 604

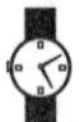

This exercise will take approximately 60 minutes to complete.

Elizabeth Washington was admitted to the ED following an automobile accident. She suffered a broken hip from the accident and has undergone an open reduction and internal fixation of the hip. She also has a history of asthma. You may have worked with Ms. Washington previously if you already completed Lesson 13 or Exercise 1 of this lesson.

- With *Virtual Clinical Excursions—Medical-Surgical* Disk 2 in your CD-ROM drive, click on the **Shortcut to VCE** icon, enter the hospital, and take the elevator to Floor 6.
- Click on the central **Nurses' Station**.
- Find and click on the **Login Computer**.
- Sign in to visit Elizabeth Washington during the 11:00–12:29 period of care.
- Listen to the Case Overview; then click on **Assignment** and read the Preceptor Note.
- Return to the Nurses' Station by clicking on the button in the bottom right corner of the screen.

- Click on **Patient Records** and select **Chart** from the drop-down menu.
- Click on **Progress Notes** and review the notes for 10:00 and 10:15.
- Return to the Nurses' Station.
- Click again on **Patient Records** and select **EPR**.
- Enter the password—**nurse2b**—and click on **Access Records**.
- Click on and review the **Vital Signs** and **Respiratory** data.

1. Ms. Washington has had an asthma attack (beginning around 10:00 a.m.) Fill in the chart below, using data from the EPR.

	10:00	10:15	10:30	10:45
Vital Signs				
BP				
HR				
RR				
SpO_2				
Respiratory				
O_2 therapy				
RUL				
RLL				
LUL				
LLL				

2. Based on your data sheet in question 1 and the information you read in the Progress Notes, answer the following questions.

   a. What physiologic change caused Ms. Washington's wheezing?

   b. What allergen likely triggered Ms. Washington's attack?

c. What would cause the increase in Ms. Washington's respiratory rate?

d. What caused an increase in her heart rate?

e. What factor resulted in a clearing of the wheezes in the RLL and LLL?

f. What caused the SpO_2 to improve by 10:30?

- To see a small-volume nebulizer, go to the Nurses' Station and click on **Patient Care**.
- Click on **Data Collection**.
- Wash your hands by first clicking in the sink and then on the faucet.
- Enter the room by clicking on the curtain on the right of the screen.
- Click on the **Chest & Back** area of the 3-D model on the left of the screen and then on each assessment option in the menu in the middle of the screen.
- Observe Ms. Washington's **Chest & Back** assessment, specifically **Respiratory Treatments.**
- Return to the Nurses' Station.
- Find and click on the MAR on the counter. Click on tab **604** to access Ms. Washington's records. Check the MAR for the use of albuterol.

3. Nebulization is a process of delivering moisture or medications into inspired air. In addition to bronchodilation, the nebulizer provided what benefit to Ms. Washington?

- Click on **Patient Records** and select **Chart** from the drop-down menu.
- Click on **Progress Notes**; once again, review the notes for 10:00.

4. Listed below are two nursing diagnoses with defining characteristics and related factors (NANDA International, 2004). Review this table and answer the questions below.

Nursing Diagnosis	Impaired gas exchange	Ineffective airway clearance
Defining Characteristics	tachycardia restlessness somnolence hypoxia dyspnea pale skin color abnormal rate of breathing	dyspnea adventitious breath sounds cough, absent cyanosis wide-eyed changes in respiratory rate
Related Factors	ventilation perfusion imbalance alveolar-capillary membrane changes	obstructed airway environmental smoking allergic airways

a. Which nursing diagnosis above most likely applies to Ms. Washington?

b. Provide a rationale for your choice.

5. For the nursing diagnosis of Ineffective airway clearance, goals of care might be to improve airflow and to relieve symptoms. Below, list two outcomes for this plan of care. Then on the next page, identify four interventions that would be appropriate for Ms. Washington's plan of care. Provide a rationale for each intervention.

Outcomes

Interventions	Rationale

6. In the list below, mark an X next to each evaluation measure that is appropriate for Ms. Washington's plan of care.

_____ a. Measure chest excursion

_____ b. Auscultate lung sounds

_____ c. Measure respiratory rate

_____ d. Ask patient to describe ease of breathing

_____ e. Palpate for fremitus

→ • Return to the Nurses' Station.

- Click on **Patient Care** and choose **Data Collection** from the drop-down menu.
- Click on **Initial Observations** and **Vital Signs** and review. Then click on the **Chest & Back** of the 3-D model and on **Respiratory** and **Respiratory Treatments** in the center menu.

7. For each of the measures used to evaluate Ms. Washington (listed below and on the next page), what were her findings upon examination?

Auscultate lung sounds

Measure respiratory rate

Ask patient to describe ease of breathing

8. Why would nasotracheal suctioning *not* be an appropriate therapy for Ms. Washington during an asthma attack?

CD-ROM Activity

Exercise 3—Tom Handy, Medical-Surgical Telemetry, Room 610

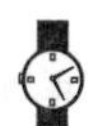

This exercise will take approximately 30 minutes to complete.

In this exercise, you will be caring for Tom Handy, a 62-year-old man admitted to the hospital for a right lobectomy for removal of a cancerous lung tumor. You may have worked with Mr. Handy previously if you already completed Lesson 15.

- With *Virtual Clinical Excursions—Medical-Surgical* Disk 2 in your CD-ROM drive, click on the **Shortcut to VCE** icon, enter the hospital, and take the elevator to Floor 6.
- Click on the central **Nurses' Station** to enter the floor.
- Find and click on the **Login Computer**.
- Sign in to care for Tom Handy at 07:00–08:29.
- Listen to the Case Overview; then click on the **Assignment** button to review the Summary of Report from your preceptor.
- Return to the Nurses' Station.
- Click on **Patient Records** and choose **Chart** from the drop-down menu.
- Review Mr. Handy's **History & Physical**.

1. According to the Assignment and Case Overview, Mr. Handy had a chest tube following surgery. A chest tube is inserted to:
   a. reestablish positive intrapleural pressure.
   b. provide an artificial airway.
   c. remove air and fluid from pleural space.
   d. remove intratracheal secretions.

2. When a chest tube accidentally becomes occluded, the patient is at risk for:
   a. tension pneumothorax.
   b. hemothorax.
   c. pulmonary emboli.
   d. subcutaneous emphysema.

3. In Mr. Handy's situation how much drainage would you normally expect in the first 24 hours after surgery? What would be the expected appearance of the fluid?

4. Care of the patient with a chest tube requires a number of precautions. Indicate whether each of the following statements is true or false.

   a. ________ A chest tube is clamped if there is an accidental disconnection of the drainage tube from the drainage collection device.

   b. ________ A patient with a chest tube draining air should be positioned on his or her side with the affected side down.

   c. ________ Any extra length of tubing can be used to allow a patient with a chest tube to stand and walk in the room.

   d. ________ Always keep the drainage system below the level at which the chest tube is inserted into the patient's chest.

   e. ________ In a water seal tube, fluid should rise with inspiration and fall with expiration.

- Return to the Nurses' Station
- Click on **Patient Care** and choose **Data Collection** from the drop-down menu.
- Wash your hands by first clicking in the sink and then on the faucet.
- Enter the room by clicking on the curtain on the right of the screen.
- Click on **Vital Signs** and on **Pain Assessment.**
- Next, click on the **Chest & Back** area of the 3-D model and on each option in the center menu. Observe each assessment.

5. Explain why it is important for Mr. Handy to cough and deep-breathe postoperatively. (*Hint:* Review Chapter 49 in your textbook.)

6. What factor increases Mr. Handy's risk for having increased pulmonary secretions postoperatively?

→ • Still within the Chest & Back assessment, click on **Respiratory** in the center menu and focus on this assessment.

7. Explain why Mr. Handy has no lung sounds over the right upper lobe.

8. Mr. Handy has a nasal oxygen cannula in place. List two complications that can develop from the use of oxygen.

9. Mr. Handy's Nursing History suggests that he may go home with oxygen. You recognize the importance of the patient managing his oxygen use safely. Based on this knowledge, a priority for Mr. Handy will be to:
   a. check the home for storage availability.
   b. locate a home care vendor for oxygen supply.
   c. learn how to check oxygen levels in tanks.
   d. stop smoking.

LESSON 12

Activity, Mobility and Skin Integrity

Reading Assignment: Activity and Exercise (Chapter 36)
Mobility and Immobility (Chapter 46)
Skin Integrity and Wound Care (Chapter 47)

Patients: Elizabeth Washington, Room 604
James Story, Room 512

Objectives

- Describe the effects of exercise on body systems.
- Describe the effects immobility has on body systems.
- Perform an assessment that identifies potential hazards of immobility for case study patients.
- Describe precautions to take for patients at risk for orthostatic hypotension.
- Determine the appropriate use of an assistive device for a patient in a case study.
- Assess a patient's risk for skin breakdown.
- Describe characteristics to observe when assessing a surgical wound.
- Describe factors that influence wound healing.
- Describe signs of wound infection.
- Identify nursing interventions designed to improve mobility.

Patients within health care settings present a wide variety of activity and mobility limitations. As a nurse, you must be able to recognize not only how patients' presenting health problems affect their ability to remain active and mobile but also how these problems pose risks for the function of all body systems. Preventive care is a key aspect of supporting a patients' mobility and activity tolerance. Early assessment is especially important as you learn to look for changes reflecting the effects of altered mobility. Application of critical thinking ensures a well thought-out plan of care that incorporates nursing interventions to keep patients active and within their limitations and to prevent complications of immobility.

A complication of immobility is impaired skin integrity. Injury to the skin poses risks to patient safety and triggers a complex healing response. Knowledge of the normal healing pattern helps a nurse recognize alterations that require intervention. This same knowledge can be applied in the care of surgical and traumatic wounds. Excellent wound care can make a significant difference in a patient's recovery and ability to return to an improved state of health.

CD-ROM Activity

Exercise 1—Elizabeth Washington, Medical-Surgical Telemetry, Room 604

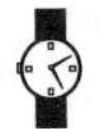
This exercise will take approximately 60 minutes to complete.

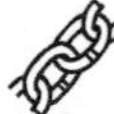
This exercise links to Lesson 11.

In this exercise you will visit Elizabeth Washington, who was admitted to the ED following an automobile accident. She suffered a broken hip from the accident and has undergone an open reduction and internal fixation of the hip. You may have worked with Ms. Washington previously.

- With *Virtual Clinical Excursions—Medical-Surgical* Disk 2 in your CD-ROM drive, click on the **Shortcut to VCE** icon, enter the hospital, and take the elevator to Floor 6.
- Click on the central **Nurses' Station**.
- Find and click on the **Login Computer**.
- Sign in to visit Elizabeth Washington during the 08:00–09:29 period of care.
- Listen to the Case Overview; then click on **Assignment** and read the Preceptor Note.
- Return to the Nurses' Station by clicking on the button in the bottom right corner of the screen.
- Click on **Patient Records** and select **Chart** from the drop-down menu.
- Review Elizabeth Washington's **History & Physical**.
- Next, click on **Operative Reports**. Review this section, specifically the Intraoperative Note.

1. The fracture of Ms. Washington's left hip was repaired with an open reduction and fixation. Initially, she was on bedrest. The temporary immobilization of the hip can result in three changes to the musculoskeletal system. Identify these changes.

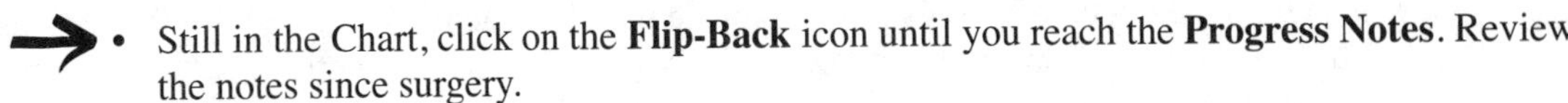

- Still in the Chart, click on the **Flip-Back** icon until you reach the **Progress Notes**. Review the notes since surgery.

2. Immobilization, even temporary, can affect a number of different body systems. Complete the chart below by reviewing the data you have for Ms. Washington. For each body system listed, check Risk or No Risk as it applies to Ms. Washington's current condition. Provide a rationale for each decision.

Body System	No Risk	Risk	Rationale
Urinary system			
Musculoskeletal			
Integument			
Metabolism			
Respiratory			

3. Based on your review of the History & Physical and Progress Notes, identify four sources of skin breakdown that apply to Ms. Washington.

4. An infection can develop in any one of the sites of skin breakdown. For each of the criteria listed below, describe the type of change associated with wound infection.

Criteria	Type of Change
Appearance of drainage	
Volume of drainage	
Skin color	
Temperature	
Comfort level	

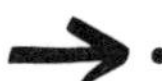

- Return to the Nurses' Station.
- Click on **Patient Care** and choose **Data Collection** from the drop-down menu.
- Wash your hands by first clicking in the sink and then on the faucet.
- Enter the room by clicking on the curtain on the right of the screen.
- Click on **Initial Observations** and observe the interaction. Next, click on **Vital Signs** and select **Pain Assessment** in the center menu. Observe the nurse's assessment of Ms. Washington's pain.
- Click on the **Upper Extremities** area of the 3-D model and observe these assessments. Then click on the **Lower Extremities** area and observe each of these assessments.

5. So far, the nurse's assessment reveals that Ms. Washington has no breakdown over pressure points. On the figure below mark an X in each circle where Ms. Washington has the highest risk for pressure based on her condition.

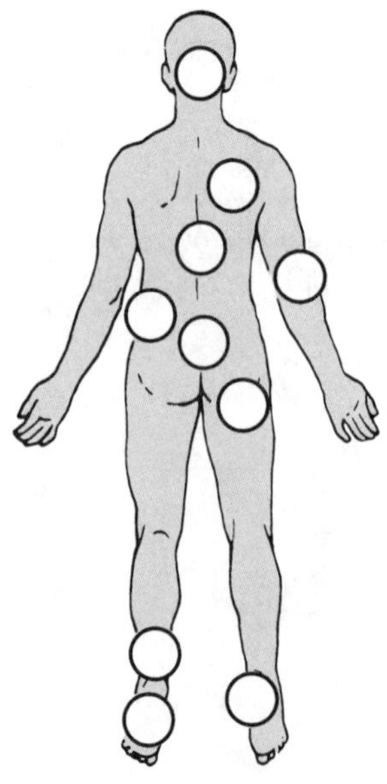

6. As the nurse assessing Ms. Washington's skin for signs of pressure, remember that she is a woman of color. Describe what an area of erythema would look like on her skin.

7. The Braden scale is used to assess a patient's risk for pressure ulcer development. Of the categories below, which do you believe apply to Ms. Washington? Provide a rationale for your answers.

Braden Category	Rationale
Sensory perception	
Moisture	
Activity	
Mobility	
Nutrition	
Friction and shear	

8. In what way would Ms. Washington's pain affect her mobility?

- Return to the Nurses' Station.
- Select **Patient Records** and click on **Kardex**. Click tab **604** to access Ms. Washington's Kardex.
- Review the outcome criteria listed in her Nursing Care Plan.

9. Ms. Washington will be using either a walker or crutches for ambulation. What factor will likely determine which of these she will use?

10. indicate whether each of the following statements describing use of crutches is true or false.

 a. ________ Handgrips of a crutch should be positioned so that the patient's body weight is supported on the axilla.

 b. ________ The length of a crutch should be three to four fingerwidths from the axilla to a point 15 cm lateral to the patient's heel.

 c. ________ Encourage patients not to lean on their crutches to support body weight.

 d. ________ The gait used for full weight bearing of both legs is the three-point gait.

 e. ________ Crutch tips should be dry and securely attached to the crutches.

11. If you were assisting Ms. Washington with her first attempt at crutch walking, list three assessments you would make to determine her activity tolerance.

12. Place an X next to each of the physiological effects of exercise.

_____ a. Increased resting heart rate

_____ b. Increased cardiac output

_____ c. Increased body heat production

_____ d. Decreased gastric motility

_____ e. Reduced alveolar ventilation

_____ f. Improved diaphragmatic excursion

→ • Return to the Nurses' Station.
- Click on to **Patient Care** and select **Data Collection**. (Remember to wash your hands before entering the patient's room.)
- Click on **Wound Condition** and observe the assessment of Ms. Washington's incision.

13. Fill in the blanks.

a. Ms. Washington's wound is healing by __________________ __________________.

b. When the edges of an incision are closed, this is called __________________________.

c. The outer edges of a wound are normally inflamed for ______________ days.

d. Serous drainage is best described as ______________________________________.

CD-ROM Activity

Exercise 2—James Story, Intensive Care Unit, Room 512

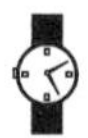

This exercise will take approximately 45 minutes to complete.

In this exercise you will visit James Story, a 42-year-old man who was admitted to the ED with symptoms of end-stage renal disease (ESRD). You may have worked with Mr. Story in a previous lesson.

- With *Virtual Clinical Excursions—Medical-Surgical* Disk 1 in your CD-ROM drive, click on the **Shortcut to VCE** icon, enter the hospital, and take the elevator to Floor 5.
- Click on the central **Nurses' Station**.
- Find and click on the **Login Computer**.
- Sign in to visit James Story during the 07:00–08:29 period of care.
- Listen to the Case Overview; then click on **Assignment**, focusing on the patient history.
- Return to the Nurses' Station by clicking on the button in the bottom right corner of the screen.
- Click on **Patient Records** and choose **Chart** from the drop-down menu.
- Click on **Nursing History**. Review the history, paying particular attention to the section on Activity and Rest.

1. Mr. Story reportedly has an occasional unsteady gait. An assessment of gait determines the status of what three functions?

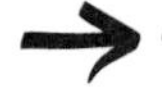

- While still in the patient's Chart, click on **Progress Notes** and read the note for Tuesday at 06:50.

2. Mr. Story has a history of being dizzy and lightheaded. He has been relatively inactive at home and has now been on bedrest since admission on Monday. This places him at risk for what condition?

3. When getting Mr. Story up for the first time, the nurse should take several precautions. Give a rationale for each of the precautions listed below.

Precaution	Rationale
Take blood pressure with patient in lying position	
Take blood pressure with patient in sitting position	
Have patient dangle on side of bed first time up	
Have staff member assist in getting patient out of bed	

4. When ambulating Mr. Story for the first time, the nurse should take what four actions to prepare the environment?

→ • Return to the Nurses' Station, click on **Patient Records**, and select **EPR**.
• Enter the password—**nurse2b**—and click on **Access Records**.
• Click on **Behavior & Activity** and review Mr. Story's ROM function.

5. The EPR reports that Mr. Story has reduced ROM in the upper right extremity. Over time any affected joints may become stiff. It will be important to coach Mr. Story through performing active ROM exercises. Indicate whether each of the following statements is true or false.

a. ________ Start any ROM exercise slowly.

b. ________ Flex the joint gently through the full range, past resistance.

c. ________ Begin exercises with proximal joints, then distal joints.

d. ________ Support the joint you are exercising distal to the joint being moved.

e. ________ During ROM assess the patient for fatigue.

→ • Return to the Nurses' Station.
• Select **Patient Care** and click on **Data Collection**.
• Wash your hands by first clicking in the sink and then on the faucet.
• Enter the room by clicking on the curtain on the right of the screen.
• Click on **Wound Condition** and observe the nurse's assessment.
• Next, click on the **Upper Extremities** area of the 3-D body model and then select each option in the center menu. Review the assessments.
• Now click on the **Lower Extremities** area of the 3-D body model and on each option in the center menu. Observe all assessments.

6. Mr. Story's arm dressing is reported to have sanguineous drainage. What does that indicate?

7. The nurse reported the size of the circle of drainage on Mr. Story's dressing as 2.5 cm in diameter. Describe an alternative to measuring the amount of drainage within a dressing.

8. Indicate whether each of the following statements describing dressing care is true or false.

a. ________ If a dry dressing adheres to the skin, pull gently to remove wound debris.

b. ________ Dressings applied to a draining wound require frequent changing.

c. ________ When removing a wet-to-dry dressing, remove the dressing once the gauze dries and pull it off to remove wound debris.

d. ________ When removing sutures, pull the visible portion of suture through underlying tissue.

9. Identify three factors from Mr. Story's history that might complicate wound healing.

LESSON 13

Elimination

Reading Assignment: Urinary Elimination (Chapter 44)
Bowel Elimination (Chapter 45)

Patients: Paul Jungerson, Room 602
Elizabeth Washington, Room 604

Objectives

- Describe factors that influence normal defecation.
- Describe factors that influence normal urination.
- Collect a nursing history of bowel elimination status of a case study patient.
- Describe factors to assess in determining the condition of an ostomy stoma.
- Describe the alterations in elimination resulting from an ostomy.
- Identify nursing interventions used to manage bowel elimination problems.
- Describe principles used in care of an indwelling urinary catheter.
- Describe nursing interventions designed to reduce the risk for urinary tract infection.
- Identify nursing interventions used to treat urinary incontinence.

CD-ROM Activity

Exercise 1—Paul Jungerson, Medical-Surgical Telemetry, Room 602

This exercise will take approximately 60 minutes to complete.

In this exercise you will visit Paul Jungerson, a retired postal worker who entered the hospital following a 3-day history of left lower quadrant pain. He had surgery Saturday for repair of a coloanal anastomosis with creation of a diverting transverse colostomy. You may have worked with Mr. Jungerson previously.

- With *Virtual Clinical Excursions—Medical-Surgical* Disk 2 in your CD-ROM drive, click on the **Shortcut to VCE** icon, enter the hospital, and take the elevator to Floor 6.
- Click on the central **Nurses' Station**.
- Find and click on the **Login Computer**.
- Sign in to visit Paul Jungerson during the 07:00–08:29 period of care.
- Listen to the Case Overview; then click on **Assignment** and review the Preceptor Note.

- Return to the Nurses' Station.
- Click on **Patient Records** and select **Chart** from the drop-down menu.
- Review the **History & Physical**
- Click on **Nursing History** and review Mr. Jungerson's history.

1. As you review Mr. Jungerson's Chart, complete the nursing history form below.

Nursing History Summary

Usual bowel elimination pattern:

Usual stool characteristics:

Routines to promote normal elimination:

Exercise:

Appetite:

Height: Weight:

Diet history:

History of surgery or illness affecting bowel elimination:

History of pain:

2. If you were the nurse caring for Mr. Jungerson, list three additional sources of data you would include in the nursing history summary.

3. Match each of the following factors with its corresponding effect on bowel elimination. (*Note:* An effect on bowel elimination may be chosen more than once.)

	Factor	**Effect on Bowel Elimination**
_____	Physical activity	a. Increases peristalsis
_____	Fluid intake less than 1000 ml daily	b. Decreases peristalsis
_____	Anxiety	c. Suppression of defecation
_____	High-fiber diet	
_____	Older adulthood	
_____	Pain	

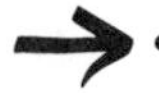

- Still in Mr. Jungerson's Chart, click on **Operative Reports**. Review this section, focusing specifically on the Report of Operation for Mr. Jungerson.

4. Mr. Jungerson has undergone a transverse colostomy. The consistency of stool effluent from the colostomy will likely be:
   a. soft formed stool.
   b. frequent liquid stools.
   c. normal solid, formed stool.
   d. water effluent

Now let's determine how Mr. Jungerson is doing following surgery.

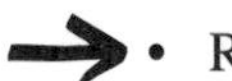

- Return to the Nurses' Station.
- Click on **Patient Care** and select **Data Collection** from the drop-down menu.
- Wash your hands by first clicking in the sink and then on the faucet.
- Enter the room by clicking on the curtain on the right of the screen.
- First, click on **Initial Observations** and view the nurse's assessment.
- Next, click on **Nutrition** and select **Oral Intake** from the center menu. After observing the video segment, select **Output** and review the assessment.
- Now click on the **Chest & Back** area of the 3-D body model, selecting **Respiratory** and **Respiratory Treatments** in the center menu.
- Finally, click on the **GI & GU** area of the 3-D model and observe the abdominal assessment by selecting each of the options in the center menu.

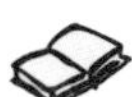

5. Mr. Jungerson is having abdominal pain and cramping. Explain how this might affect his breathing. (*Hint:* Review Chapter 49 in your textbook.)

6. Evaluate the physical examination findings for Mr. Jungerson by writing "Normal" or "Abnormal" next to each description below.

   a. ______________ Abdomen is large and round.

   b. ______________ Stoma red and moist.

   c. ______________ Bowel sounds hypoactive.

   d. ______________ Stool from stoma is liquid.

7. List three characteristics of an effective ostomy pouching system.

→ • Still in the Data Collection screen, observe the appearance of Mr. Jungerson's stoma one more time (*Hint:* Click on **Nutrition**, then on **Output**).

8. For each of the assessment measures listed below, provide a rationale.

Assessment Measure	Rationale
Assess stoma shape and presence of swelling	
Observe condition of skin barrier and pouch	
Observe abdominal incision	
Inspect condition of skin around stoma	

→ • Return to the Nurses' Station.
- Click on **Patient Records** and select **Chart** from the drop-down menu.
- Click on **Progress Notes**. Read the Postoperative Progress Notes, specifically the entry for Monday at 18:40.

9. Mr. Jungerson will be learning how to care for his colostomy once he returns home. Suppose he were to say, "I have a neighbor who had a colostomy. He says he used to always put an aspirin in the pouch to control odor. He also told me that he had trouble doing the activities he enjoyed. The pouch always leaked." What would be your response to Mr. Jungerson?

10. Identify whether each of the following statements is true or false.

   a. ________ During the first weeks following surgery, Mr. Jungerson will likely be on a high-fiber diet.

   b. ________ Foods such as broccoli, cauliflower, and dried beans may cause gas and odor.

   c. ________ Bathing the skin around an ostomy without proper drying can cause skin breakdown.

   d. ________ Cold drinks are effective in stimulating peristalsis.

CD-ROM Activity

Exercise 2—Paul Jungerson, Medical-Surgical Telemetry, Room 602

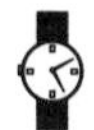

This exercise will take approximately 30 minutes to complete.

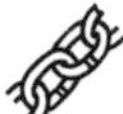

This exercise links to Lesson 9.

In this exercise you will visit Paul Jungerson, a retired postal worker who entered the hospital following a 3-day history of left lower quadrant pain. He had surgery Saturday for repair of a coloanal anastomosis with creation of a diverting transverse colostomy. You may have worked with Mr. Jungerson previously in Exercise 1. If you are continuing directly from Exercise 1, sign out from your current period of care and log in again to work with Mr. Jungerson for the 07:00–08:29 period of care. If you are just starting for the day and do not already have the software running, follow the steps below:

- With *Virtual Clinical Excursions—Medical-Surgical* Disk 2 in your CD-ROM drive, click on the **Shortcut to VCE** icon, enter the hospital, and take the elevator to Floor 6.
- Click on the central **Nurses' Station**.
- Find and click on the **Login Computer**.
- Sign in to visit Paul Jungerson during the 07:00–08:29 below.
- Listen to the Case Overview; then click on **Assignment** and review the Preceptor Note.
- Return to the Nurses' Station.
- Click on **Patient Records** and select **Chart** from the drop-down menu.
- Click on **Physician Orders** and review the orders for Saturday at 16:15.

1. Mr. Jungerson has an order for an indwelling Foley catheter to be inserted postoperatively. It was likely inserted during surgery. What is the purpose of the indwelling catheter in this situation? (*Study Tip:* Review Chapter 49 of your textbook.)

- Return to the Nurses' Station.
- Click on **Patient Records** and select **EPR** from the drop-down menu.
- Enter the password—**nurse2b**— and click on **Access Records**.
- Review the data collected for Monday in the following areas: **GI & GU**, **Drains & Tubes**, and **Intake & Output**.

2. Complete the assessment summary below for Mr. Jungerson's data from Monday.

Data Summary
24-hour intake from Monday 00:01 to 23:59:
24-hour output from Monday 00:01 to 23:59:
Character of urine:
Condition of Foley:
Foley care:

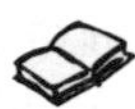

3. Are Mr. Jungerson's 24-hour intake and output normal or abnormal? (*Study Tip:* Review normal I&O in Chapter 40 in your textbook.)

4. What is the most common complication that can develop from an indwelling catheter insertion?

5. With the development of a urinary tract infection, the character of the urine is likely to become:
   a. bloody.
   b. dark amber in color.
   c. foamy.
   d. cloudy and thick.

6. On the diagram below, place an arrow at the points where infectious organisms can enter the sterile urinary tract to cause infection.

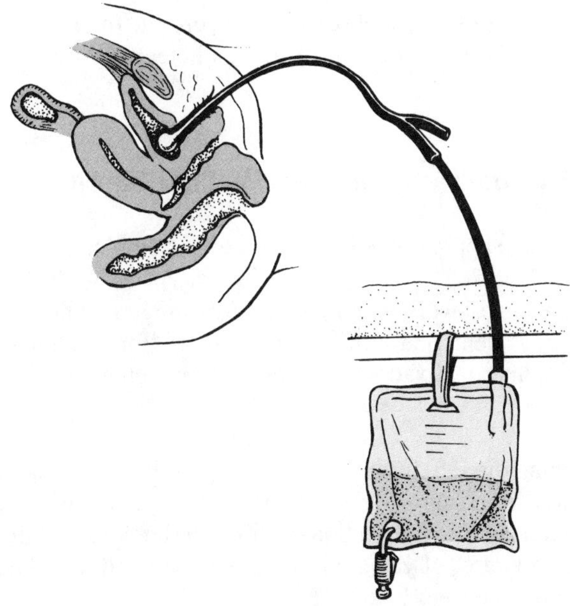

7. Consider the procedure for providing indwelling catheter care. Match each of the steps below with its corresponding rationale.

	Step	Rationale
_____	Place patient in supine position.	a. Reduces secretions likely to contain microorganisms
_____	Retract foreskin.	b. Ensures access to perineal tissues
_____	Ask patient whether burning or discomfort is felt.	c. Moves from area of least contamination to most
_____	Spread urethral meatus and cleanse around catheter, then around meatus.	d. Permits inspection of meatus for inflammation and discharge
_____	Use soap and water to wipe along length of catheter.	e. Determines presence of infection

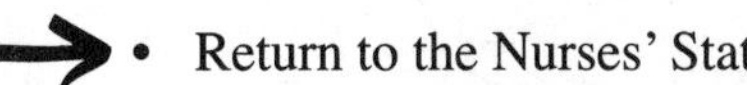

- Return to the Nurses' Station.
- Click on **Patient Records** and select **Chart**.
- Click on **Physician Orders** and review the orders for Monday at 19:10.

8. Mr Jungerson is to have his Foley catheter removed. Identify whether each of the following statements is true or false.

a. ________ Insert a syringe with needle into injection port to withdraw fluid from the balloon.

b. ________ Normally a patient will feel burning as the catheter is withdrawn.

c. ________ It is unusual for the patient to have urinary retention after the catheter removal.

d. ________ If a patient fails to void 8 hours after catheter removal, it may become necessary to reinsert a catheter.

e. ________ A nurse must observe and record the time and the amount of urine passed with the first voiding after catheter removal.

CD-ROM Activity

Exercise 3—Elizabeth Washington, Medical-Surgical Telemetry, Room 604

This exercise will take approximately 30 minutes to complete.

For this exercise, you will work with Elizabeth Washington, who was admitted to the ED following an automobile accident. She suffered a broken hip from the accident and has undergone an open reduction and internal fixation of the hip. You may have worked with Ms. Washington previously.

If you are continuing directly from Exercise 1, sign out from your current period of care and log in to work with Ms. Washington, for the 09:00–10:29 period of care. (*Note:* If you need help, see p. 27 of the **Getting Started** section of this workbook for detailed steps on switching patients or periods of care.) If you are just starting for the day and do not already have the software running, follow the steps below:

- With *Virtual Clinical Excursions—Medical-Surgical* Disk 2 in your CD-ROM drive, click on the **Shortcut to VCE** icon, enter the hospital, and take the elevator to Floor 6.
- Click on the central **Nurses' Station**.
- Find and click on the **Login Computer**.
- Sign in to visit Elizabeth Washington during the 09:00–10:29 period of care.
- Click on to the **Assignment** and review the Case Overview.
- Return to the Nurses' Station.
- Click on **Patient Records** and select **Chart** from the drop-down menu.
- Click on **Progress Notes** and review the notes for Monday at 06:30.
- Click on **Physician Orders** and read the order for 06:30 on Monday.

Ms. Washington has an order to discontinue the Foley catheter Monday. To assess how well she tolerates removal of the catheter, review the EPR.

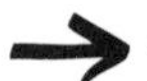

- First, return to the Nurses' Station; then click on **Patient Records** and select **EPR**.
- Next, enter the password—**nurse2b**—and click on **Access Records**.
- Click on **Intake & Output** and review data.

1. Record the following data based on your EPR review.

Volume of urine at first voiding:

Time of first voiding:

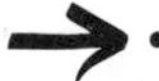

- Return to the Nurses' Station.
- Click on **Patient Care** and choose **Data Collection** from the drop-down menu.
- Wash your hands by first clicking in the sink and then on the faucet.
- Enter the room by clicking on the curtain on the right of the screen.
- Click on the **Behavior** button and then on **Activity** in the middle of the screen. Observe the video.
- Click on the **GI & GU** area (abdomen) of the 3-D model.
- One at a time, click on each additional option in the middle of the screen to observe the complete assessment.

2. What was the condition of Ms. Washington's urine at the first voiding, and what level of activity is she assuming?

3. With Ms. Washington's activity still limited, she may require a bedpan for voiding. Which of the following describes the correct approach for placing Ms. Washington on a bedpan?
   a. Position patient supine with head of bed flat; have her plant both feet on mattress and lift her hips as you slip bedpan into place. Keep bed flat.
   b. Have Ms. Washington use the overhead trapeze to lift herself up as the bedpan is positioned under her.
   c. In supine position, elevate patient's head 30 degrees; have her plant both feet on mattress and lift her hips as you slip bedpan into place.
   d. Position patient flat and have her roll to side; place bedpan against buttocks and have patient roll back onto plan. Keep bed flat.

4. Match each urinary alteration with its corresponding description.

	Description	Urinary Alteration
_____	Diminished capacity to form urine	a. Polyuria
_____	Discomfort during urination	b. Diuresis
_____	Inability to produce urine	c. Oliguria
_____	An excessive output of urine	d. Anuria
_____	Increased urine formation	e. Dysuria

- Return to the Nurses' Station.
- Click on **Patient Records** and select **Chart** from the drop-down menu.
- Review Ms. Washington's Nursing History.

5. Ms. Washington's history reveals that she takes the medication hydrochlorothiazide and drinks decaffeinated coffee and tea regularly. What effect do these two factors have on urination.

6. Ms. Washington's history also reveals that she passes urine when she laughs too hard. This is likely a symptom of:
   a. urge incontinence.
   b. reflex incontinence.
   c. overflow incontinence.
   d. stress incontinence.

7. Fill in the blanks:

   a. Ms. Washington's incontinence problem would likely improve through use of

      ____________________ exercises.

   b. A sudden increase in ____________________ pressure commonly causes stress incontinence.

   c. The best time of day to take a diuretic is ____________________.

   d. A patient with stress incontinence should never ignore the urge to

      ____________________.

   e. Two methods used to initiate voiding are ____________________ and

      ____________________.

LESSON 14

Care of the Surgical Patient

Reading Assignment: Care of Surgical Clients (Chapter 49)

Patient: Darlene Martin, Surgery and PACU, (Floor 4); Medical-Surgical Telemetry, Room 613

Objectives

- Identify patient's risks for postoperative complications.
- Explain the factors related to physiologic responses to surgery.
- Assess a postoperative patient's status following surgery.
- Identify nursing diagnoses pertinent to patients in the case studies.
- Discuss rationale for use of clinical interventions for patients in the case studies.
- Evaluate effect of postoperative interventions.

Perioperative nursing care includes nursing care given before (preoperative), during (intraoperative), and after surgery (postoperative). Throughout the course of a patient's surgical experience, a nurse learns to make thorough and comprehensive assessments, comparing the patient's preoperative baseline with postoperative measurements. Effective and efficient patient assessment ensures that appropriate surgical interventions are selected. For example, understanding a patient's risk for complications preoperatively allows a nurse to take measures to prevent complications postoperatively. A surgical patient can often be an active participant in care by learning and performing postoperative exercises, reporting any unusual symptoms or sensations that can indicate problems, and by following any postoperative restrictions. Together, the nurse and patient can make the surgical experience uneventful and ensure a patient's return to normal function as soon as possible.

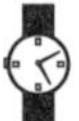

CD-ROM Activity

Exercise 1—Darlene Martin, Surgery (Floor 4)

This exercise will take approximately 60 minutes to complete.

- With *Virtual Clinical Excursions—Medical-Surgical* Disk 2 in your CD-ROM drive, click on the **Shortcut to VCE** icon, enter the hospital, and take the elevator to Floor 4.
- When you arrive at Floor 4, click on the central **Nurses' Station**.
- Find and click on the **Login Computer**.
- Sign in to visit Darlene Martin during the Preop Interview.

- Listen to the Case Overview; then click on **Assignment** and read the Preceptor Note. Be sure to answer the questions posed in the Case Overview.

The first step in providing appropriate care of a surgical patient is to collect a thorough and relevant nursing history.

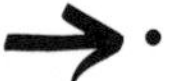

- Click on **Nurses' Station** in the lower right of the screen.
- Click on **Patient Records** and then select **Chart** from the drop-down menu.
- Read the **History & Physical**; then click on **Nursing History** and review this section also.

Complete the following worksheet.

Preoperative VS:

BP _______ HR _______ RR _______ Temp _______ PaO_2 _______

Weight: Height:

Cardiovascular function:
Apical HR: Heart sounds:

Skin color and temperature:

Elimination function:

Nutrition/metabolic function:
Eating patterns:

Perception and cognition:

Self-perception:

Sexuality:

Past experience with surgery:

1. Based on your review of Ms. Martin's history, how would you classify her surgery?
   a. Minor palliative
   b. Major elective
   c. Reconstructive
   d. Major urgent

2. After a review of Ms. Martin's History & Physical and Nursing History, list any risk factors you believe may increase her risk during the surgical experience. Explain how each risk factor might affect the patient.

3. A surgical patient who has history of nausea following anesthesia is at risk for:
   a. negative nitrogen balance.
   b. infection.
   c. aspiration.
   d. atelectasis.

→ • Continue to review Ms. Martin's preoperative database by clicking on **Laboratory Reports** and reviewing her test results.

4. It is important to check all laboratory values on Ms. Martin before she goes to surgery. Record her results from the Laboratory Reports below.

WBC

Hemoglobin

Hematocrit

Potassium

Sodium

Glucose

5. a. What is the reason for measuring Ms. Martin's hemoglobin and hematocrit?

   b. What is the normal value for WBC in an adult?

   c. If the WBC count were above normal, what would Ms. Martin be at risk for?

d. Identify one intervention commonly used to manage sodium and potassium levels during surgery.

- Return to the Nurses' Station.
- Click on **Patient Care**. Click on **Case Overview** and listen to the report.
- Return to the Nurses' Station.
- Click on **Patient Care** and choose **Data Collection** to go to Ms. Martin's room.
- Wash your hands by first clicking in the sink and then on the faucet.
- Enter the room by clicking on the curtain on the right of the screen.
- Click on the **Initial Observations** button and watch the video.

6. Now that you have reviewed Ms. Martin's Nursing History and observed the nurse's initial observations, list two facts you know about the patient that should be incorporated into your approach for preoperative teaching.

   a.

   b.

7. Match each postoperative exercise step with its rationale.

	Postop Exercise Step	**Rationale**
_____	Have patient take slow, deep breaths, inhaling through nose.	a. Allows for gradual expulsion of air.
_____	Instruct patient to place palms of hands across from each other, down and along lower borders of anterior rib cage.	b. Allows patient to feel movement of chest and abdomen as diaphragm descends and lungs expand.
_____	Instruct patient to avoid using chest muscles while inhaling.	c. Reduces useless energy expenditure.
_____	Have patient hold slow, deep breath for count of 3 and then slowly exhale through pursed lips.	d. Prevents panting or hyperventilation.

8. Ms. Martin is asked to turn and reposition following surgery. What do you know about her condition preoperatively that might affect her ability to turn effectively?

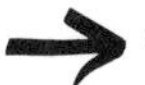

- Return to the Nurses' Station
- Click on **Planning Care** and select **Problem Identification** from the drop-down menu.

9. Listed in the right column below are four possible nursing diagnoses that might apply to Ms. Martin, especially postoperatively. Match each nursing diagnosis with its defining characteristics. (*Note:* Each diagnosis will have more than one defining characteristic.)

	Defining Characteristics	**Nursing Diagnosis**
_____	Expresses an interest in learning	a. Anxiety
_____	Increased swallowing	b. Readiness for enhanced knowledge
_____	Altered chest excursion	c. Nausea
_____	Uncertainty	d. Risk for ineffective breathing pattern
_____	Depth of breathing <500 ml tidal volume	
_____	Relates previous experience pertaining to topic	
_____	Report of nausea	
_____	Apprehension	

CD-ROM Activity

Exercise 2—Darlene Martin, Surgery (Floor 4)

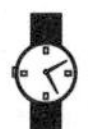

This exercise will take approximately 45 minutes to complete.

If you are continuing directly from Exercise 1, sign out from your current period of care and log in again to work with Ms. Martin, this time for the 06:30–7:29 period of care. (*Note:* If you need help, see p. 27 of the **Getting Started** section of this workbook for detailed steps on switching patients or periods of care.) If you are just starting for the day and do not already have the software running, follow the steps below:

- With *Virtual Clinical Excursions—Medical-Surgical* Disk 2 in your CD-ROM drive, click on the **Shortcut to VCE** icon, enter the hospital, and take the elevator to Floor 4.
- When you arrive at Floor 4, click on the central **Nurses' Station**.
- Find and click on the **Login Computer**.
- Sign in to care for Darlene Martin, this time during Preoperative Care, 06:30–07:29.
- Listen to the **Case Overview**; then click on **Assignment** and review the Preceptor Note.
- Return to the Nurses' Station.
- Click on **Patient Care** and select **Data Collection**. (Remember to wash your hands.)
- Once you enter the patient's room, click on **Initial Observations**. Review the initial findings.
- Then click on **Vital Signs** and review the patient's preoperative baseline vital signs.

Record Ms. Martin's baseline vital signs below:

BP __________ HR __________ RR __________ T __________ PaO_2 __________

- Continue your review of Ms. Martin's assessment by clicking on the **Head & Neck** area of the 3-D model.
- Click on each of the additional options and observe each area of the assessment.

1. Explain what the Head & Neck assessment fails to cover that is important in a preoperative review.

- Click on the **Chest & Back** area of the 3-D model and observe each of those assessments.

2. a. Complete the diagram below, mapping out the stethoscope placement for where the nurse actually assessed Ms. Martin's lung sounds. Enter the sequence of numbers in the proper blanks. (*Study Tip:* Review Chapter 32 in your textbook.)

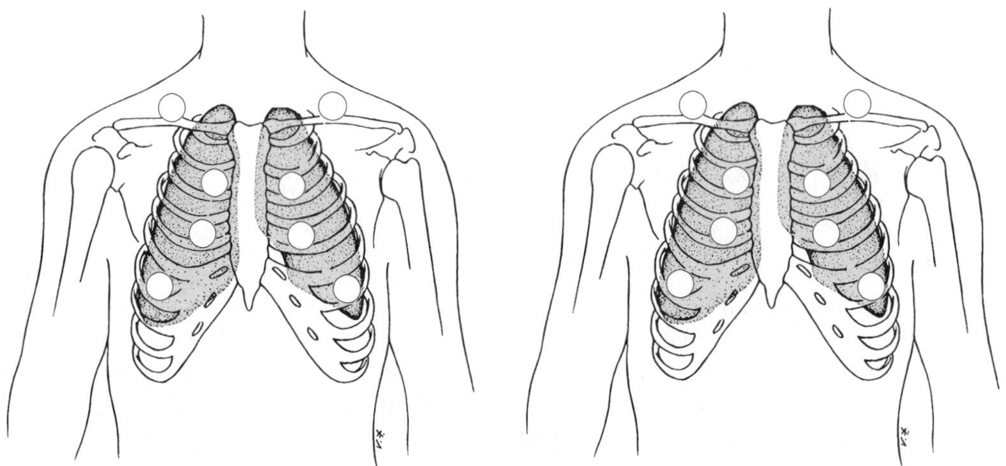

Ideal auscultation pattern | Actual auscultation pattern

b. Did the nurse use an appropriate technique? Explain.

3. The nurse's assessment of the patient's lung sounds would have been better if the patient had been:
   a. positioned on her side.
   b. asked to breathe through the nose with mouth closed.
   c. sitting upright with arms forward.
   d. lying supine in bed.

- Click on the **GI & GU** area of the 3-D model and review each assessment in the center menu.

4. The assessment reveals that Ms. Martin's bowel sounds are normal and active in all four quadrants. What bowel sounds findings would you expect postoperatively? Explain.
   a. Active
   b. Absent
   c. Hyperactive

- Click on the **Lower Extremities** of the 3-D model and review each assessment in the center menu.

5. Record the following findings from Ms. Martin's Lower Extremities assessment.

Vascular

Integumentary

6. Considering what you know about Ms. Martin's history and after reviewing a description of an abdominal hysterectomy (*Hint:* Review description in your medical dictionary), vascular assessment provides a baseline for determining what complication postoperatively?
   a. Hemorrhage
   b. Pulmonary embolus
   c. Thrombus
   d. Hypoxemia

7. What is the rationale for a patient to perform foot and leg exercises postoperatively?

- Click on **Nutrition** on the left side of the screen; then click on **Parenteral Intake**.

8. The patient has an IV of lactated Ringer's running at ________ ml/hr. Calculate the drip rate (gtt per minute), assuming that the IV infusion set delivers 10 gtt/ml. (*Hint:* Refer to Chapter 40 in your textbook.)

- Click on **Behavior** on the left side of the screen.
- Review each assessment in the center menu.

9. Return to p. 172 of this lesson and review the findings from your initial review of Ms. Martin's Nursing History, specifically her self-perception, sexuality, and past experience with surgery. Then consider what you observed when the nurse assessed Ms. Martin's behavior. Describe your impressions in each of the following categories. (*Hint:* Refer to you textbook, pp. 1603–1604.)

Emotional health

Body image

Coping resources

- Return to the Nurses' Station.
- Click on **Patient Records** and select **Chart**.
- Click on **Physician Orders**. Review the orders written by the surgeon.

10. Match each of the following physician's orders with its rationale.

	Physician's Order	Rationale
_____	NPO	a. Adjunct for induction of anesthesia
_____	Foley catheter insertion	b. Reduces risk for wound infection
_____	Droperidol IV	c. Prevents risk for gastrointestinal upset, including postop nausea and vomiting
_____	Gentamycin IV	d. Promotes bladder emptying

11. Current scientific recommendations for preoperative fasting suggest that patients fast from intake of clear liquids for:
    a. 12 hours before surgery.
    b. 2 to 3 hours before surgery.
    c. 6 or more hours before surgery.
    d. 24 hours before surgery.

- Still in Ms. Martin's Chart, click on **Operative Reports**.

12. Ms. Martin is known to be allergic to penicillin and ampicillin, two antibiotics. It is also important to find out whether a surgical patient has a latex allergy. Place an X next to each item below that may contain latex.

_____ Thermometer sheath

_____ Gloves

_____ IV tubing

_____ Sphygmomanometer cuff

_____ Foley catheter

CD-ROM Activity

Exercise 3—Darlene Martin, PACU (Floor 4)

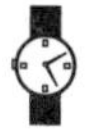

This exercise will take approximately 30 minutes to complete.

If you are continuing directly from Exercise 2, sign out from your current period of care and log in again to work with Ms. Martin in the PACU for the 09:30 period of care. (*Note:* If you need help, see p. 27 of the **Getting Started** section of this workbook for detailed steps on switching patients or periods of care.) If you are just starting for the day and do not already have the software running, follow the steps below:

- With *Virtual Clinical Excursions—Medical-Surgical* Disk 2 in your CD-ROM drive, click on the **Shortcut to VCE** icon, enter the hospital, and take the elevator to Floor 4.
- When you arrive at Floor 4, click on the central **Nurses' Station**.
- Find and click on the **Login Computer**.
- Listen to the **Case Overview**; then click on **Assignment** and review the Preceptor Note.
- Return to the Nurses' Station.
- Click on **Patient Records** and choose **Chart** from the drop-down menu.
- Click on **Operative Reports** and read Ms. Martin's records.

1. After reviewing the data in Ms. Martin's records, complete the following information.

   a. Patient's position on the OR table:

   b. Location of grounding pad:

   c. Method of restraint:

   d. Were antiembolism stockings applied?

   e. Urinary output in PACU:

   f. Oral intake in PACU:

   g. Complication during surgery:

2. Surgical patients are at risk for perioperative position injury. Indicate whether each of the following statements is true or false.

   a. ________ In an anesthetized patient, perception of joint position is increased.

   b. ________ In an anesthetized patient, muscles are very relaxed.

   c. ________ During surgery, patients' positions are changed frequently.

   d. ________ Patients placed in unusual positions are aligned anatomically to reduce pressure on the skin.

3. Why it is significant to know that Ms. Martin had ice chips in the PACU?

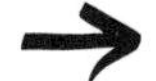

- Return to the Nurses' Station.
- Click on **Patient Care** and choose **Data Collection** from the drop-down menu.
- Wash your hands by first clicking in the sink and then on the faucet.
- Enter the room by clicking on the curtain on the right of the screen.
- Click on **Initial Observations** and then on **Vital Signs**.
- Review Ms. Martin's initial assessment and her PACU vital signs.

4. Compare Ms. Martin's preoperative vital signs (recorded on the top of p. 176) with her vital signs in the PACU. Your conclusion of her status is:
   a. BP has increased slightly with pulse and temperature stable.
   b. Heart rate is more irregular with slight hypotension.
   c. BP has decreased slightly, heart rate is stable, and she remains hypothermic.
   d. Oxygen saturation is falling with a slight decrease in BP.

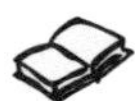

5. Explain why Ms. Martin's BP has dropped slightly and her pulse has increased. (*Hint:* Review Table 49-10 in your textbook.)

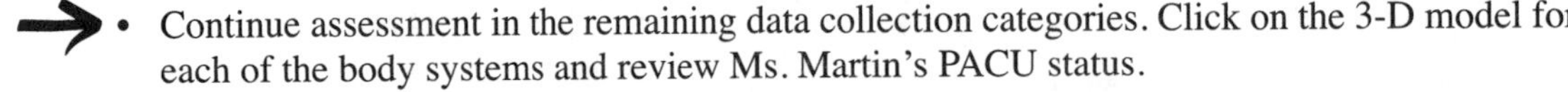

- Continue assessment in the remaining data collection categories. Click on the 3-D model for each of the body systems and review Ms. Martin's PACU status.

6. If you compare the assessment of Ms. Martin's respiratory status in the PACU with the preoperative holding area (see question 2), what difference do you notice?

7. List three factors that might influence Ms. Martin's ability to take a deep breath.

8. It will be important for Ms. Martin to begin use of an incentive spirometer as soon as possible. Number the following steps in the correct order.

_____ Have patient repeat maneuver until goals are achieved.

_____ Be sure she places the mouthpiece of the spirometer so that her lips completely cover the mouthpiece.

_____ Have patient sit in semi-Fowler's position.

_____ Ask patient to inhale slowly and maintain constant flow through the unit, attempting to reach goal volume. Have her hold her breath for 2 to 3 seconds and then exhale slowly.

_____ Set on the spirometer scale the volume level to be attained with each breath.

_____ Instruct patient to breathe normally for short period and then repeat maneuver.

9. After observing the assessment of the patient's integument, how would you critique the nurse's approach? What would you do differently?

10. The wound assessment reveals that Ms. Martin has serosanguineous drainage on her dressing. Is this normal?

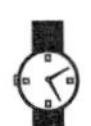

CD-ROM Activity

Exercise 4—Darlene Martin, Medical-Surgical/Telemetry Floor, Room 613

This exercise will take approximately 45 minutes to complete.

- With *Virtual Clinical Excursions—Medical-Surgical* Disk 2 in your CD-ROM drive, click on the **Shortcut to VCE** icon, enter the hospital, and take the elevator to Floor 6.
- Click on the **Nurses' Station** to enter the floor.
- Locate the Login Computer and sign in to care for Darlene Martin in Room 613 at 11:00–12:29.
- Listen to the **Case Overview** and read the Assignment.
- Return to the Nurses' Station.
- Click on **Patient Records** and choose **MAR** from the drop-down menu.
- Click on tab **613** to access Ms. Martin's records. Compare the information you learned in the assignment overview with information in the MAR.

1. Fill in the blanks:

   The nurse reports that the patient received __________ mg of morphine sulfate and that Ms. Martin's pain rating was reduced from ______ to ______. The MAR record shows that the patient received __________ mg of morphine sulfate at 10:00 and __________ mg of morphine sulfate at 11:00.

2. What inconsistency exists in the above data? What would you do?

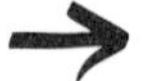

- Return to the Nurses' Station.
- Click on **Patient Care** and choose **Data Collection** from the drop-down menu.
- Wash your hands by first clicking in the sink and then on the faucet.
- Enter the room by clicking on the curtain on the right of the screen.
- Click on the **Vital Signs** button on the left of the screen.
- Review the assessment of the patient's vital signs, specifically the **Pain Assessment**.

3. a. How has Ms. Martin's self-report of pain changed since she was in the PACU? (*Hint:* Also review her pain ratings in the EPR.)

   b. As the nurse, what would you do?

4. What pain relief method might be more effective for Ms. Martin? (*Hint:* In Chapter 42 of your textbook, review the section on Pharmacologic Pain Relief Interventions.)

- Click on the **Chest & Back** area of the revolving 3-D model. Then click on each assessment option in the menu in the middle of the screen. Review all assessments.

5. Findings in the musculoskeletal category show that Ms. Martin's skin is pale. This is most likely due to:
   a. the effects of sedatives.
   b. the fact that her skin was already pale preoperatively.
   c. the effects of pain.
   d. blood loss, which causes anemia.

- Click on the **GI & GU** portion of the 3-D model. Then click on each button in the menu in the middle of the screen. Review all assessments.
- Click on **Wound Condition** and review the assessment.

6. List two methods for assessing the amount of wound drainage from a surgical wound.

- Click on **Nutrition** and then on each option in the center menu. Review all assessments.
- Return to Nurses' Station.
- Click on **Patient Records** and select **Chart** from the drop-down menu.
- Click on **Progress Notes** and review.
- Return to the Nurses' Station and click on **Patient Records**.
- This time, choose **EPR** from the drop-down menu. (*Remember:* The password is **nurse2b**.)
- Read the EPR, specifically the **Hygiene** section.

7. Ms. Martin has been able to eat ice chips. She tells the nurse her mouth is dry. What intervention would you, as the nurse, initiate?

8. Ms. Martin is progressing well from her surgery. To fully evaluate her recovery status, you must apply a critical thinking model. Complete the following diagram by writing the letter of each critical thinking factor under its corresponding category.

Knowledge

(1) ___________

(2) ___________

(3) ___________

Experience

(4) ___________

Evaluation of Surgical Condition

Standards

(5) ___________

(6) ___________

(7) ___________

Attitudes

(8) ___________

Critical Thinking Factors

a. Refer to the Infusion Nurses Society Standards for Phlebitis.
b. Demonstrate perseverance in having patient perform postop exercises.
c. Consider time spent previously caring for patient with colon resection.
d. Signs and symptoms of common postoperative complications.
e. Use established expected outcomes to evaluate patient's response to therapies.
f. Review the physiologic responses to stress of surgery.
g. Consider behaviors that demonstrate learning.
h. Use accurate observational measures (e.g., pain score).

LESSON 15

Loss and Grief and Nursing Interventions to Support Coping

Reading Assignment: The Experience of Loss, Death, and Grief (Chapter 29)
Stress and Coping (Chapter 30)

Patients: Julia Parker, Room 608
Tom Handy, Room 610

Objectives

- Describe loss and the grief responses that patients experience.
- Distinguish among the types of loss.
- Explain the relationship between loss and stress.
- Identify characteristics of a person experiencing grief.
- Describe coping mechanisms used by patients in the case studies.
- Develop a nursing plan of care for a patient experiencing grief.
- Apply the critical thinking model to a patient experiencing grief.

Loss and grief are experiences that commonly affect the patients you care for. It is important for a patient to be able to express grief and to feel the pain associated with a loss in order to achieve healing. Grief affects an individual physically, psychologically, socially, and spiritually. For example, grief can trigger the stress response, causing a number of physiologic, emotional, and intellectual responses. A nurse's role is to assist a patient to feel a loss and to complete the tasks of the grief process. One way to assist is by understanding a patient's normal coping resources and to promote interventions that enhance the patient's hope, self-esteem, dignity, and expression of grief.

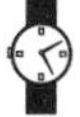

CD-ROM Activity

Exercise 1—Julia Parker, Medical-Surgical Telemetry, Room 608

This exercise will take approximately 60 minutes to complete.

- With *Virtual Clinical Excursions—Medical-Surgical* Disk 2 in your CD-ROM drive, click on the **Shortcut to VCE** icon, enter the hospital, and take the elevator to Floor 6.
- Click on the **Nurses' Station** to enter the floor.
- Find the Login Computer and sign in to care for Julia Parker at 07:00–08:29.
- Listen to the **Case Overview** and click on the **Assignment** to read the Preceptor Note.

- Return to the Nurses' Station.
- Click on **Patient Records** and select **Chart** from the drop-down menu.
- Review the Nursing History, paying special attention to the Self-Perception, Role Relationships, Coping and Stress Tolerance, and Life Principles sections.
- Return to the Nurses' Station.
- Click on **Patient Care** and select **Data Collection**.
- Wash your hands by first clicking in the sink and then on the faucet.
- Enter the room by clicking on the curtain on the right of the screen.
- Click on the **Behavior** button, then on each additional option in the center menu.
- Observe the nurse's assessment of the patient's Behavior.

1. Describe the type of loss Ms. Parker has suffered through each of the following experiences. Give a rationale for your answers.

Death of her husband

Her own heart attack

2. Match each of the following descriptions of Ms. Parker's behavior with its corresponding behavior type.

	Description	Behavior Type
_____	Patient is frightened; says she feels like a "cardiac cripple."	a. Mourning
		b. Bereavement
_____	Looks for information to understand what might have caused heart attack.	c. Grief
_____	Patient is unable to accept loss of injury to her heart and feels a need at times to express anger.	

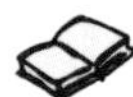

3. Nursing care of a grieving patient begins with establishing a caring presence and determining the significance of the patient's loss. What therapeutic communication strategies did the nurse use in assessing Ms. Parker's signs of distress? What communication approaches were perhaps less effective? (*Hint:* Refer to Chapter 23 in your textbook for help.)

4. Julia Parker is obviously experiencing a significant loss. To more fully assess her grief response, you must apply a critical thinking approach. Complete the diagram below by writing the letter of each critical thinking factor under its corresponding category.

Knowledge

(1) ___________

(2) ___________

(3) ___________

Experience

(4) ___________

(5) ___________

Assessment of Grief Response

Standards

(6) ___________

(7) ___________

(8) ___________

Attitudes

(9) ___________

Critical Thinking Factors

a. Allow Ms. Parker to give a complete account of the concerns she has about her heart attack.
b. If you have cared for a patient who has suffered a life-threatening illness, apply what you learned in assessing Ms. Parker.
c. Review the theories of grief and the stages of the grief process.
d. Allow Ms. Parker to decide whether and how to involve her family and clergy person in your assessment of her needs.
e. Know the effects of a myocardial infarction on heart function.
f. Ms. Parker has shown an uncertainty over her future. Approach the assessment by helping her to discuss what is relevant to her.
g. Apply what you have learned about the importance of relationships with close family members.
h. Ms. Parker was a clinical psychologist before retirement. Approach the assessment by asking her how she has helped others who have experienced loss.
i. Consider the role of the family in coping.

5. Identify whether each of the following statements pertaining to theories of grief is true or false.

a. ________ A person progresses through the stages of grief or mourning in a linear fashion.

b. ________ According to Worden, it is common for a person to not realize the full impact of a loss for at least 3 months.

c. ________ Bowlby's phase of numbing is similar to Kübler-Ross's stage of depression.

d. ________ During reorganization, a person adapts to unaccustomed roles and acquires new skills.

- Review once again Ms. Parker's discussion of her concerns with the nurse. Still in her room, click on **Behavior** and on the additional options as needed to answer question 6.

6. In the list below, mark an X next to the symptoms of normal grief that Ms. Parker exhibited.

   _____ Disorganization

   _____ Anxiety

   _____ Confusion

   _____ Acceptance

   _____ Self-reproach

- Return to the Nurses' Station
- Click on **Patient Records** and select **Chart**.
- Click on **Nursing History** and review again.

7. Discuss each of the following factors that influence the grief response as they pertain to Ms. Parker.

Spiritual beliefs

Personal relationships

Nature of the loss

Socioeconomic status

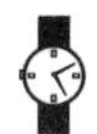

CD-ROM Activity

Exercise 2—Julia Parker, Medical-Surgical Telemetry, Room 608

This exercise will take approximately 45 minutes to complete.

In this exercise you will visit Julia Parker. She is a 51-year-old patient who was admitted to the ED with symptoms of a heart attack (myocardial infarction). You may have worked with Ms. Parker previously if you already completed Lesson 1.

If you are continuing directly from Exercise 1, sign out from your current period of care and log in again to work with Ms. Parker, this time for the 09:00–10:29 period of care. (*Note:* If you need help, see p. 27 of the **Getting Started** section of this workbook for detailed steps on switching patients or periods of care.) If you are just starting for the day and do not already have the software running, follow the steps below:

- With *Virtual Clinical Excursions—Medical-Surgical* Disk 2 in your CD-ROM drive, click on the **Shortcut to VCE** icon, enter the hospital, and take the elevator to Floor 6.
- Click on the **Nurses' Station**.
- Find and click on the **Login Computer**.
- Sign in to care for Julia Parker at 09:00–10:29.
- Listen to the **Case Overview**.
- Return to the Nurses' Station.
- Click on **Patient Records** and select **Chart** from the drop-down menu.
- Click on **Nursing History** and review this section.
- Now click on **Physician Orders** and review the MD orders for Sunday at 07:45 for an emergency.
- Next, click on **Progress Notes** and review.

1. If Ms. Parker reported feeling anxious and noted a tightness in her chest along with an increase in blood pressure, how might you determine whether this was a response to stress or whether she was having a worsening myocardial infarction? What action would you take?

2. Match each dimension of hope with its corresponding nursing strategy.

	Dimension of Hope	Nursing Strategy
_____	Affective dimension	a. Focus on short-term goals.
_____	Affiliative dimension	b. Reminisce about achievements or positive moments in life.
_____	Contextual dimension	c. Reinforce expressions of positive thinking and realistic goal setting.
_____	Temporal dimension	d. Encourage patient to foster relationships with family.

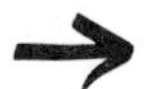

- Return to the Nurses' Station.
- Click on **Patient Care**; then select **Data Collection**. (Remember to wash your hands.)
- Click on **Initial Observations** and then on **Behavior**. Select each of the behavior categories in the center menu and review the assessments.

3. The nurse says to Ms. Parker, "I tell you what, we are going to do an EKG, draw blood, and get something for pain. After the results get back, we will be able to tell what is going on." In what way is this statement therapeutic? (*Hint:* Review what you learned from Ms. Parker's Nursing History.)

You are ready to consider a nursing diagnosis and create a care plan for Ms. Parker. To identify a priority nursing diagnosis, review all you have learned from the behavioral assessments of the patient during this lesson. (*Hint:* Review the patient's behaviors for both the 07:00–08:29 and 09:00–10:29 periods of care.) Consider what you observed during your most recent visit with Ms. Parker (above), as well as her responses to the nurse in Exercise 1 (p. 186).

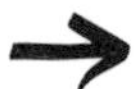

- Return to the Nurses' Station.
- Click on **Planning Care**; then select **Setting Priorities** from the drop-down menu.
- Click on the **Nursing Case Matrix** at the bottom of the screen and review the nursing diagnosis information.

4. Ms. Parker presents data suggestive of the nursing diagnosis Anxiety. Develop a care plan for her using the form on the next page. Choose the assessment characteristics that best fit Ms. Parker's situation from what you have observed in the behavioral assessments. Then identify two outcomes that are most suited to her situation. Finally, for each outcome, select suggested interventions most appropriate for Ms. Parker.

Nursing Care Plan

Nursing Diagnosis:

Assessment Characteristics:

Outcomes	Suggested Interventions
1.	
2.	

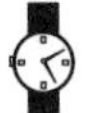 **CD-ROM Activity**

Exercise 3—Tom Handy, Medical-Surgical Telemetry, Room 610

This exercise will take approximately 30 minutes to complete.

In this exercise, you will be caring for Tom Handy, a 62-year-old man admitted to the hospital for a right lobectomy for removal of a cancerous lung tumor. You may have worked with Mr. Handy previously if you already completed Lesson 15.

If you are continuing directly from Exercise 1 of this lesson, switch patients by logging out and signing in to work with Tom Handy at 07:00–08:29 on the Login Computer (see p. 27 in the **Getting Started** section for help). If you are just starting for the day and do not already have the software running, follow the steps below:

- With *Virtual Clinical Excursions—Medical-Surgical* Disk 2 in your CD-ROM drive, click on the **Shortcut to VCE** icon, enter the hospital, and take the elevator to Floor 6.
- Click on the central **Nurses' Station**.
- Find and click on the **Login Computer**.
- Sign in to visit Tom Handy at 07:00–08:29.
- Listen to the **Case Overview**; then click on **Assignment** and review the Preceptor Note.
- Go to the Nurses' Station.
- Click on **Patient Records**; then select **Chart**.
- Click on **Nursing History** and review.

1. Hospitalization poses a number of losses for Mr. Handy. In the list below, mark an X next to those losses most likely to apply to him.

   _____ Loss of control over body function

   _____ Threat to independence

   _____ Threat to ability to perform his job

   _____ Change in role that his wife assumes in his care

   _____ Loss of ability to make decisions

- Return to the Nurses' Station.
- Click on **Patient Care**; then select **Data Collection**. (Remember to wash your hands.)
- Click on the **Behavior** button and then on each option in the center menu.
- Review the Behavior assessments.

2. Describe the type of grief Mr. Handy is experiencing and provide a rationale to your answer.

3. Match each type of grief with its corresponding description.

	Description	Type of Grief
_____	Active acute mourning that does not subside and continues over long periods of time	a. Anticipatory grief
		b. Delayed grief
_____	Grief in which person does not recognize that behaviors interfering with normal functioning are a result of loss	c. Masked grief
		d. Chronic grief
_____	The process of "saying good-bye" before an actual loss	
_____	Suppressed or postponed expression of grief	

4. Complete the following data sheet, describing what you have learned about Mr. Handy in each of these areas of assessment.

a. Mr. Handy's type of loss is:

b. Phase of grief (Bowlby):

Assessment of Factors Influencing Grieving

c. Personal relationships:

d. Spiritual beliefs:

e. Human development:

f. Influence on personal lifestyle:

LESSON 16

Self-Concept

Reading Assignment: Self-Concept (Chapter 26)

Patients: James Story, Room 512
James Franklin, Room 504

Objectives

- Identify components of self-concept.
- Describe stressors affecting the self-concept of patients in the case studies.
- Discuss the influence family members have on patients' self-concept.
- Describe approaches used to assess a patient's self-concept.
- Apply critical thinking in developing a plan of care for a patient who has an altered self-concept.
- Discuss a patient in a case study who has resources to support a positive self-concept.

The self-concept is a complex mixture of thoughts, attitudes, and perceptions that shape how a person thinks about himself or herself. A person's self-concept consequently affects a person's self-esteem, how one feels about himself or herself. Throughout life numerous factors play a role in developing, nurturing, and threatening a person's self-concept. The associated stresses of illness and disability are no exception. As a nurse it is important for you to know that a person's self-concept influences his or her perception of health and thus the ability to cope with illness and assume healthy behaviors. You can play an important role in helping patients adapt to stressors and to use the resources they have in maintaining or restoring their self-concept.

CD-ROM Activity

Exercise 1—James Story, Intensive Care Unit, Room 512

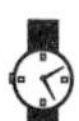

This exercise will take approximately 60 minutes to complete.

In this exercise you will visit James Story, a 42-year-old man who was admitted to the ED with symptoms of end-stage renal disease (ESRD). You may have worked with Mr. Story previously if you already completed Lesson 7 or 9.

- With *Virtual Clinical Excursions—Medical-Surgical* Disk 1 in your CD-ROM drive, click on the **Shortcut to VCE** icon, enter the hospital, and take the elevator to Floor 5.
- Click on the **Nurses' Station** to enter the floor.
- Find and click on the **Login Computer**. Sign in to care for James Story the 07:00–08:29 period of care.

- Listen to the **Case Overview**; then click on **Assignment** and review the Preceptor Note, focusing on the patient history.
- Return to the Nurses' Station.
- Click on **Patient Records** and choose **Chart** from the drop-down menu.
- Click on **Nursing History** and review.

1. James Story suffers serious chronic disease. As you review the Nursing History, what stressors can you identify in the following four categories that have potentially influenced Mr. Story's self-concept?

Body image

Role performance

Self-esteem

Identity

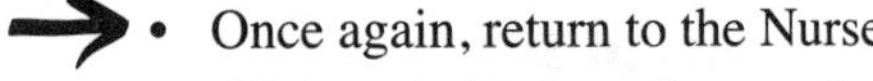

- Once again, return to the Nurses' Station.
- Click on to **Patient Care** and select **Data Collection**.
- Wash your hands by first clicking in the sink and then on the faucet.
- Enter the room by clicking on the curtain on the right of the screen.
- Click on the **Behavior** button on the left of the screen.
- Select each of the subcategories in the center menu to observe the complete assessment of Mr. Story's behavior.

2. After observing the behavioral assessment, what additional stressors affecting Mr. Story are you able to identify?

3. The best description of self-concept is:
   a. a person's self-appraisal of relationship with other individuals.
   b. the roles an individual assumes in life.
   c. a person's perception of his or her body.
   d. a combination of factors that provides a sense of wholeness and consistency.

4. The family influences the development of one's self-concept. Identify two family factors that may have played a role in Mr. Story's self-concept development.

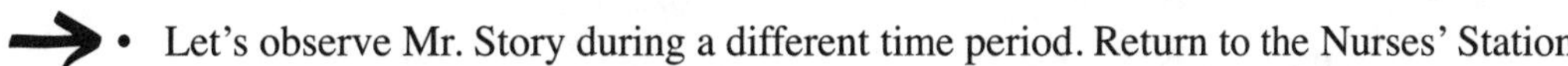

- Let's observe Mr. Story during a different time period. Return to the Nurses' Station.
- Find and click on the **Login Computer**.
- Click on the **Supervisor's Computer** button and then return to the Nurses' Station. This logs you out of the current time period.
- Click on the **Login Computer** again and sign in to care for Mr. Story at 11:00–12:29.

5. Match each role performance stressor with its corresponding description.

	Role Performance Stressor	Description
_____	Role conflict	a. Mr. Story feels frustrated and inadequate in his role as a husband.
_____	Role ambiguity	b. When employed, Mr. Story had difficulty balancing his time and energy as an employee and as a patient in the sick role.
_____	Role strain	c. Because of Mr. Story's chronic illness, he must attend to numerous responsibilities, including taking multiple medications, going to dialysis, following treatment restrictions.
_____	Role overload	d. When faced with multiple illnesses and associated symptoms, Mr. Story "does not know what's happening." Expectations of him are unclear.

6. Mr. Story reveals a great deal during the behavioral assessment. However, the nurse could explore even more with the patient. For each of the following components, list an assessment question to explore Mr. Story's self-concept more fully.

Self-Concept Components	Assessment Question
Self-esteem	
Role	
Identity	

- Now, let's observe Mr. Story during the 09:00–10:29 period of care.
- Return to the Nurses' Station.
- Find and click on the **Login Computer**.
- Click on the **Supervisor's Computer** button and then return to the Nurses' Station.
- Click on the **Login Computer** again and sign in to care for Mr. Story at 09:00–10:29.
- Return to the Nurses' Station.
- Click on **Patient Care** and choose **Data Collection** from the drop-down menu. (Remember to wash your hands before entering the patient's room.)
- Click on the **Behavior** button on the left of the screen and on each additional option in the center menu.

7. Part of your assessment of a patient's self-concept includes observation of nonverbal behaviors. In the list below, place an X next to each behavior you observed in Mr. Story.

a. _____ Overly critical

b. _____ Avoidance of eye contact

c. _____ Negative self-evaluation

d. _____ Difficulty in making decisions

e. _____ Hesitant speech

8. Mr. Story's case reveals numerous nursing diagnoses. For the nursing diagnosis of Disturbed body image, match each of the following defining characteristics with Mr. Story's corresponding behavior.

	Defining Characteristic	Mr. Story's Behavior
_____	Verbalization of feelings that reflect an altered view of one's body.	a. "I stopped doing that a long time ago. Just hanging around the house."
		b. "Tired of dialysis and being sick."
_____	Actual change in body function	
		c. "I just want to feel normal."
_____	Change in social involvement	
		d. Has peripheral neuropathy with loss of sensation in extremities.
_____	Verbalization of change in lifestyle	
_____	Negative feelings about body	e. "I don't have many friends."

9. As you consider developing a plan of care for Mr. Story, demonstrate how you would apply critical thinking by writing the letter of each critical thinking factor under its corresponding correct category below.

Knowledge

(1) ___________

(2) ___________

(3) ___________

Experience

(4) ___________

Planning Mr. Story

Standards

(5) ___________

(6) ___________

Attitudes

(7) ___________

Critical Thinking Factors

a. The time you have spent caring for patients with body image disturbances will assist you in planning care for James Story.
b. Apply principles of therapeutic communication as you select approaches to strengthen Mr. Story's coping behaviors.
c. Maintain Mr. Story's dignity as you plan to discuss options for ways to help him become more productive.
d. Mr. Story is a complex patient. Show humility in what you do not know and seek suggestions for his care plan from a social worker.
e. Review components of self-concept in determining types of interventions for the plan of care.
f. In planning care, be complete when summarizing data about Mr. Story's relationship with his wife so that you can include her as an appropriate resource.
g. Consider principles of caring as you form your relationship with Mr. Story.

10. For each of the following goals of care, write an outcome statement:

Goal	Outcome Statement
Mr. Story will identify and express feelings about his physical illness by day of discharge.	
Mr. Story will identify a sense of control over his medical treatment within 48 hours.	
Mr. Story will identify resources available to him outside the hospital by discharge.	

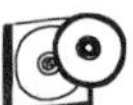

CD-ROM Activity

Exercise 2—James Franklin, Intensive Care Unit, Room 504

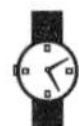

This exercise will take approximately 45 minutes to complete.

In this exercise you will visit James Franklin, a 67-year-old man who underwent a right carotid endarterectomy following several episodes of transischemic attacks. You may have worked with Mr. Franklin previously if you already completed Lesson 17.

- With *Virtual Clinical Excursions—Medical-Surgical* Disk 1 in your CD-ROM drive, click on the **Shortcut to VCE** icon, enter the hospital, and take the elevator to Floor 5.
- Click on the **Nurses' Station** to enter the floor.
- Find and click on the **Login Computer**.
- Log in to visit James Franklin during the 07:00–08:29 period of care.
- Listen to the **Case Overview**; then click on **Assignment** and review the Preceptor Note.
- Return to the Nurses' Station.
- Click on **Patient Records** and choose **Chart** from the drop-down menu.
- Click on **Nursing History** and review Mr. Franklin's history.

1. Mr. Franklin is 67 years of age. His success in achieving an age-appropriate stage of self-concept development is crucial. After reviewing his Nursing History, describe Mr. Franklin's status in each of the following areas.

Sense of competency

Academic- and employment-related identity

Spiritual identity

Current feelings about physical self

Personal relationships

2. Older adults have unique self-concept stressors. What is most likely Mr. Franklin's greatest self-concept stressor?

3. If you already completed Lesson 1, you learned about Mr. Story, a victim of chronic disease. His self-concept stressors are listed below. (*Study Tip:* Go to Lesson 1 and review Mr. Story's Nursing History.) Mr. Franklin's clinical picture is somewhat different and offers an interesting comparison when reviewing self-concept principles. For each type of stressor identified for Mr. Story below, describe the corresponding stressor for Mr. Franklin.

Mr. Story's Stressor	Mr. Franklin's Stressor/resource
Identity: Engages in minimal socialization; a husband who is unable to perform sexually	Identity:
Role performance: Limited financial resources, unemployed	Role performance:
Self-esteem: Robbed of a healthy life	Self-esteem:
Body image: Reduced energy and vision; multiple chronic diseases	Body image:

4. Mr. Franklin's Nursing History reveals that he wants to active be active and vital and that he is prepared to follow a plan to prevent a stroke. List three interventions that might be useful in supporting his self-concept.

5. Indicate whether each of the following statements is true or false.

a. ________ A person's role performance may develop from imitation, the acquisition of knowledge and skills from other members of one's social group.

b. ________ A patient in his mid-20s to mid-40s has a self-concept developmental task of showing contentment with age.

c. ________ Low self-esteem in college age women has been associated with depression.

d. ________ An older adult who becomes preoccupied with physical complaints may have an unhealthy self-concept.

LESSON 17

Principles Applied in Care of Older Adults

Reading Assignment: Older Adult (Chapter 13)

Patient: James Franklin, Room 504

Objectives

- Identify common myths about older adults.
- Describe developmental tasks of older adults.
- Identify physical findings of patients in the case studies that can be influenced by physiological changes of aging.
- Describe psychosocial changes of aging.
- Describe common health concerns of an older adult.
- Explain how principles of gerontology influence selection of nursing interventions.

American society is getting older. The number of older adults in the United States is growing in proportion to the total population. As a nurse, it is important for you to understand that every older adult is unique in the way he or she adjusts to aging. The nursing care of older adults is challenging because of the great variation in patients' physiological, cognitive, and psychosocial health. Older adults also vary widely in their levels of functional ability. Most older adults are very active and involved with their families and communities. A smaller number have lost the ability to care for themselves and are unable to make decisions concerning their daily needs. Principles of gerontologic nursing help you to apply the nursing process in an age-appropriate way to meet the needs of your older adult patients.

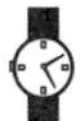

CD-ROM Activity

Exercise 1—James Franklin, Intensive Care Unit, Room 504

This exercise will take approximately 75 minutes to complete.

In this exercise you will visit James Franklin, a 67-year-old man who underwent a right carotid endarterectomy following several episodes of transischemic attacks. You may have worked with Mr. Franklin if you completed Lesson 16.

- With *Virtual Clinical Excursions—Medical-Surgical* Disk 1 in your CD-ROM drive, click on the **Shortcut to VCE** icon, enter the hospital, and take the elevator to Floor 5.
- Once you have entered the Nurses' Station and accessed the Login computer, sign in to visit James Franklin during the 07:00–08:29 period of care.

- Listen to the **Case Overview**; then click on **Assignment** and review the Preceptor Note.
- Click on the **Nurses' Station** button in the lower right corner of the screen.
- Click on **Patient Care** and select **Data Collection**.
- Inside Mr. Franklin's room, click on the **Vital Signs** button and then on each assessment option in the menu in the middle of the screen.
- Next, click on the appropriate areas of the 3-D body model to observe the nurse's assessment of Mr. Franklin's status in the following areas: **Head & Neck**, **Chest & Back**, **GI & GU**.

1. Listed below are findings from Mr. Franklin's assessment. In the right-hand column fill in common physiological changes associated with aging for each finding.

Mr. Franklin's Assessment Findings	Physiologic Changes of Aging
PERRLA	
Hearing within normal limits	
Is able to inhale more than 2500 ml using incentive spirometer	
BP 109/71	
Bowel sounds normoactive	
Voids spontaneously	

- Continue your Data Collection by clicking on **Initial Observations** and observing the interaction.

2. While assessing Initial Observations, the nurse used communication techniques suited to older adults. List three appropriate techniques used by the nurse.

3. Mr. Franklin initially appears to be a healthy older adult. There are many myths or stereotypes about older adults that can influence their nursing care. Indicate whether each of the following statements is true or false.

   a. ________ A normal older adult retains interest in sexual activities.

   b. ________ The majority of older adults live in institutional settings.

   c. ________ Most older adults have old-fashioned notions and are not open to new ideas.

   d. ________ An older adult normally has difficulty acquiring new knowledge.

   e. ________ Many older adults hold an optimistic view of life and retain broad social contacts.

- Click on the **Nurses' Station** button in the lower right corner of the screen. Wash your hands by clicking in the sink and then on the faucet. Click on the door to leave the area.
- Click on **Patient Records** and select **Chart** from the drop-down menu.
- Click on **Nursing History** and review Mr. Franklin's history.

4. As you review Mr. Franklin's history, note the entries describing his interest in learning about stroke prevention. Fill in the blanks in the following statements describing approaches to support older adults' learning.

   a. To ensure that an older patient understands what you have explained, ask for

      ____________________.

   b. To help older patients concentrate on learning, focus discussion on a single

      ____________________.

   c. When speaking to an older adult, it is helpful to keep the tone of voice _____________.

   d. To help a patient like Mr. Franklin learn about a stroke, you might provide verbal instruction but then offer ________________ cues in the form of drawings.

5. All older adults face certain developmental tasks. The way an older adult adjusts to these tasks is very individualized. For each of the developmental tasks listed below, describe the corresponding behavior Mr. Franklin has assumed.

Developmental Task	Mr. Franklin's Behavior
Adjusting to death of a spouse	
Finding ways to maintain quality of life	
Adjusting to diminishing health	
Maintaining satisfactory living arrangements	

6. Refer to what you have learned in the textbook about assessment of psychosocial changes in older adults. For each factor below, describe what you would like to assess more fully in the case of Mr. Franklin.

Retirement

Relationship with family members

Housing

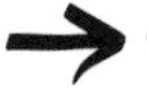

- Still within the Nursing History in the Chart, review the medications Mr. Franklin has been taking at home.
- Click on the **Nurses' Station** button in the lower right corner of the screen.
- Find the MAR on the counter.
- Click on to the **MAR** to review Mr. Franklin's current medications. (Remember to click on Mr. Franklin's room number—**504**—to access the correct records.)

7. An older adult's sexual functioning may be impaired by use of:
   a. antihypertensives.
   b. diuretics.
   c. antibiotics.
   d. antipyretics.

8. Many older adults take numerous medications to manage both acute and chronic medical conditions. What is the greatest risk posed by polypharmacy?

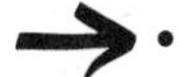

- Click on the **Nurses' Station** button in the lower right corner of the screen.
- Click on **Patient Records** and select **Kardex**. Click on tab **504** (Mr. Franklin's room number) and review the nursing diagnoses and problems selected for him.
- Again, click on the **Nurses' Station** button in the lower right corner of the screen.
- Click on **Patient Care**; this time select **Data Collection**. (Remember to wash your hands.)
- Click on **Initial Observations** and observe the interaction.
- Click on **Behavior** and then select **Activity**.

9. Mr. Franklin is identified as being at risk for neurologic deficit. Specifically, there is concern that despite his surgery, he may be at risk for having another transischemic attack. Fall prevention will be an important nursing intervention. In the list below, place an X next to each fall risk factor that is applicable to Mr. Franklin (*Study Tip:* Consider what you have observed in the patient data collection and previous MAR data. Also check the EPR for additional information on Mr. Franklin's current status.)

   _____ a. Is receiving a sedating medication

   _____ b. Has episodes of disorientation

   _____ c. Equipment such as intravenous tubing and wires from monitors that pose obstacles to safe ambulation

   _____ d. Is at risk for orthostatic hypotension

   _____ e. Has impaired vision

- Continue the Data Collection by clicking on the 3-D model's **Chest & Back** area. Click on **Respiratory** and then on **Respiratory Treatments** in the center menu to focus on these assessments.

10. Another nursing diagnosis identified for Mr. Franklin is *Risk for infection*. Identify the reason for older adults to be at risk for nosocomial infection in the hospital.

11. After reviewing the Data Collection on Mr. Franklin, the nurses are focused on preventing which of the following nosocomial infections?
    a. Surgical wound infection
    b. Bloodstream infection
    c. Urinary tract infection
    d. Pneumonia

12. Mr. Franklin is among those older adults at risk for having a stroke. The Healthy People 2010 initiatives address health promotion programs for older adults. List three Healthy People 2010 elements of health promotion that would apply to Mr. Franklin.

Notes

Notes

Notes

Notes

Notes